Jamba Juice® Power

Jamba Juice® Power

smoothies and juices
for mind, body,
and spirit

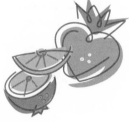

Kirk Perron
Founder of Jamba Juice®

with Stan Dembecki

AVERY
A MEMBER OF PENGUIN GROUP (USA) INC.
NEW YORK

AVERY

a member of
Penguin Group (USA) Inc.
375 Hudson Street
New York, NY 10014
www.penguin.com

Library of Congress Cataloguing-in-Publication Data

Perron, Kirk.
    Jamba Juice power! : smoothies and juices for mind, body, and spirit / by Kirk
Perron with Stan Dembecki.
        p.   cm.
    Includes bibliographical references and index.
    ISBN 1-58333-177-8
        1. Fruit juices—Therapeutic use.   2. Smoothies (Beverages).   3. Blenders (Cookery).
    4. Fruit—Therapeutic use.   5. Exercise   6. Health   I. Dembecki, Stan.   II. Title.
    RM237.P47   2004   2003057755
    641.3'4—dc22

Printed in the United States of America
10   9   8   7   6   5   4   3   2

This book is printed on acid-free paper. ∞

Book design by Lovedog Studio

Spot art © Jamba Juice® Company

For the full Jamba experience, visit your local Jamba Juice store.

To my partner, Lou Lou (Louis)

And my family: Chur Mah, my mom; Laura Fay, my twin sister; Jimmy (James Jeffrey Poppleton), my beloved brother-in-law who should be in marketing, thanks for all the ideas; Todd, my brother; Teresa, my sister-in-law; and Nicholas, my nephew

And to my dad, Lloyd: You will live on in our hearts forever.

Contents

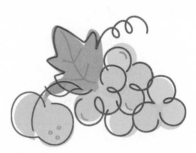

Acknowledgments

One of the most important ingredients that goes into every smoothie we serve here at Jamba is the effort of our dedicated team members. It is because of their vast storehouses of energy and help that we have been able to build Jamba into the quality brand that it is today . . . all of which has been done one smoothie at a time.

Of course, Jamba would never have come as far as it has without the solid foundation and unlimited supply of dedication, imagination, and good old-fashioned hard work put in place by my noble friends and founding Juice Club team members. I wish to express deep thanks to the spirited and classy Kevin Peters for helping to create the best-operating system in the business; Joe Vergara for patiently teaching me everything there was to know about how to properly operate a smoothie and juice store; and Linda Olds for her endless support and keen marketing intuition. Who would have guessed way back when that we kids, most in our early twenties, would one day amount to such a great team? Wow.

I always knew I wanted to start a business of my own someday and luckily back at high school in Morro Bay, California, my English teacher took me under her wing and taught me the basics of how to do just that. Thank you, Mrs. Carrie Martini, for believing in me, and for giving all of your students the courage to follow their dreams. You are truly an angel.

I'd also like to give particular thanks and acknowledgment to others who have helped me in more ways than they'll ever know: Ed Collar, Michael Wilhelm, Trevor Sanders, Michael Hieshima, Gina Kerr, Jen

Morehouse, Gloria Thompson, Allison Baughman, Patrick Baughman, Andrea Doorack, Steve Marko, Jim Worster, John Greiner, and Sukari (Georgia) Addison. (Yo, John and Sukari, we still have that wine to drink. Don't forget!)

Today, our success is entirely due to the dedication and dynamic leadership of Paul Clayton. Paul, Jamba would not be in the leadership position today without you. I can't thank you enough for all of your hard work and commitment to making Jamba into one of the world's truly meaningful and magnificent brands. It is thanks also to the rest of the leadership team—Joe O'Neil, Lynne McFarlane, Karen Kelley, Renee Kempler, Jason Walthall, Rhondi Shigemura, Thad Logan, Mark Eddy, Rosa Compean, Bonnie El Halta, Anne Kimball, Kent Lansville, Maureen Tramontana, Steve Adkins, Jason Briscoe, Henry Hirschel, Greg Pick, Michael Perun, and Kevin Wilkinson—that Jamba is able to shine as brilliantly as it currently does.

I want to send a warm and heartfelt message of gratitude to my beautiful mother, Lea Perron, for her remarkable support and unconditional love. Thank you, Bob West and Mom, for helping me get the first store started by loaning me part of the necessary funds. I will never forget the help and assistance you provided me in my time of need.

Thanks also: Sue Felt, Matt Collar, Joe Vergara, and Felton Ferrini, for helping to bridge the gap between success and possible ruin in those early days before we were able to stand on solid ground and begin to grow from the efforts of venture financing. You are all truly amazing.

Speaking of the past, I'm not sure if Jamba Juice would be here today if Roy Domenghini and John Guidetti hadn't put in a good word for me with Felton Ferrini, our first landlord, who asked them for references into my character. Thanks, Felton, for taking that risk on an energetic kid like me, and for all your support, advice, and help along the way. I simply couldn't have done it without all you!

One of our first franchisees likes to say, "You built the rocket, but I launched it!" To you, Robert McCormick, a special note of gratitude goes out from the bottom of my heart for taking the risk and opening the second store, or launching the rocket, if you will. Yes, you did it. Also, a hearty thanks goes to: Celia Denig and Scott Graeber, Robert and Charlotte McCormick, Errol and Margo Bisutti, Judi Munley and Dick Munley, Trevor Kensey, Larry Appell, Jeff Wilson and Dean Kahn, Mary Schock and Mark Keenan, Brian and Katie Howard, Matt Boyd, Bill and Miles Littell, David Sester and Lyndell Campbell, and to all our other franchisees, for pouring your hearts and souls into transforming our stores into the great successes that they are known as today.

From the very start, here at Jamba we have believed in the philosophy of striving to be the best, and without the significant investment in our infrastructure we would never have been able to grow as effectively and quickly as we did. I am especially grateful to Bob Kagle of TVI and Benchmark Capital (Bob, thanks for believing in me, even when I didn't); Craig Foley of Whickham Capital; Jamie Shennan of Trinity Ventures; Howard Goldstein of Invesco; Jerry Gallagher of Oak Investment Partners; Cece Smith of Philips-Smith, Kyle Anderson and Chip Adams of Rosewood Capital; and all the other individual investors who have helped over the years.

For proudly serving on our board of directors and bringing a hands-on perspective to our team, thank you: John Mackey and Howard Schultz. Without your patience, steadfast vision, and extraordinary support, Jamba would never have been able to come as far.

In addition, I'd like to offer sincere thanks to the following highly valued people, who poured their blood, sweat, and tears into making our vision for Jamba become a reality: Chris Baer, Jim Mizes, Michael Keller, Bob Andrews, Rene Boer, Tom Hough, Silva Raker, Glenn Bacheller, Chris Strausser, Julia Scocimara, David Whisenhunt, Joe David, Bill McCarthy, Lorraine Morton-Feazell, John Powers, David Rich, Dede Hilovsky, Sue Webb, Mara Meisner, Susan Sablan, Mark Archer, Manoj Tripathi, and Ray Miolla.

Getting the right location is half of the equation in making our stores a success, so thank you Michael Epsteen, Tina Essegian, Nancy Johnson, and all of the other brokers, landlords, property managers, and agents who have worked to secure great real estate. Sincere thanks also go out to Ken Smith, Nita Smith, and all the other distributors for partnering with us to get our product into as many stores as possible.

Rich Maire, Susan Hollander, Vince Waldman, David Holmes, Michael Joblove, and Ziyad Naccasha, thank you for all your expert legal advice. Jack Anderson, Lisa Cerveny, and the rest of the Hornall Anderson design team, thank you for creating our phenomenal logo and terrific graphic identity. Richard Altunas, Howard Backon, and Keith Smith, thanks for your great store designs. Jeff Smith, Jill Sandin, and all of our other PR partners around the country, thanks for helping get the word out about Jamba. Thanks also to Alice Elliott, John Plummer, and our other dedicated recruiters for helping to build an amazing team. Eric Flamholtz, thanks for your keen planning ideas and development expertise. Thanks: Pete Mattson and your entire team for your imaginative product ideas; Butler, Shine and Stern and Mad Dogs and Englishmen for all the cool Jambaisms; Bill Peters and Blane Peters for your risk management advice; and Mike Doherty and Tony Garland (I love you, guys!), thanks for your much-needed financial help and more than anything, your friendship. Also to Gabe McCauley for helping to keep my life organized. And to Dr. Charles Spezzano and the Fruit Goddess (Laura Lee Garcia), for sparking the idea that I could write a book.

I'd also like to send out a very special thank-you to our Wellness Advisory Board: Sue Havala Hobbs, Ph.D., M.S., R.D., Mitchell May, Dr. Lee Lipsenthal, Todd Harrison, and Dave Scott, for your passion, your efforts, your expertise, and for sharing your vast knowledge with us.

To our agent, Mary Ann Naples, at the Creative Culture, thank you for believing that we could actually write this book and for realizing its potential to help people. Thanks also go to: Susan Pepper for your expertise in sorting out our troubles regarding this book's proposal. Thank you, Dr. Sue Havala Hobbs and Dr. Lee Lipsenthal, for carefully reviewing and offering your critical comments. I realize that neither of you agrees with every word I have written. To John Duff, Eileen Bertelli, and the rest of the happy, healthy, sexy staff at Avery/Penguin for your belief, support, and enormous help with this book and all the legal entwinements that needed to be sorted out to make it possible.

And an exceptionally special thank-you goes to my coauthor, Stan Dembecki, for working tirelessly (and for many months without pay), even when many doors seemed closed, to make this book a great one. Stan, you're the best!

In closing, I'd like to acknowledge all our customers who have been the fuel for what we do. And to Aleah, one of our very first customers, who seemed a bit cranky in the beginning, who we later found out had been suffering from the ravages of cancer, whom every team member grew to love as her final months faded away: Your spirit will live on in our hearts forever.

Foreword

Do you want to be healthier, happier, and fitter? Of course you do.

For years I've been coaching my patients on wellness and disease prevention. I've been urging people to eat a balanced diet that includes plenty of fresh fruits and vegetables. I've encouraged people to get more out of life by learning to love themselves, and not just by taking care of their physical well-being, but by carefully attending to their emotional and spiritual self as well. Fortunately, I finally have a place for them to turn to for gentle, well-guided support . . . Welcome to the awesome pages of *Jamba Juice® Power: Smoothies and Juices for Mind, Body, and Spirit,* featuring a perfectly blended 21-Day Lifestyle Plan to nourish your body, refresh your mind, and boost your spirit— *for life*—written by the visionary founder of Jamba Juice, Kirk Perron.

After all, becoming healthier and happier is only as difficult as we allow it to be. We live on an earth that has abundant resources. We are surrounded by beauty and opportunity. Look at the spectacular plants around you, the fantastic foods, and smell the fresh air. The next time you are at a lake appreciate that this is a healthy resource in an incredible package! Our fruits and vegetables are also remarkable packages, made by nature for our pleasure and health. Look at those around you, wonderful, interesting people with whom you can share years of pleasure, also in an incredible array of interesting packages.

While you're enjoying life to the fullest with people you love the most, turn back to Mother Nature anytime you may need help. Begin savoring the joys of natural foods that make sense. Fruits, vegetables, fish, legumes, and other low-fat, high-fiber foods and whole-wheat grains from a significant variety of sources have consistently been shown, in scientific literature, to prevent and aid treatment of multiple health problems; the short list includes: heart disease, diabetes, many cancers, osteoporosis, high blood pressure, and obesity. Importantly, the list also includes depression, anxiety, hostility, attention deficit disorder, and other states of emotional distress. Yes, food affects mood!

So dive into Kirk's refreshing new program and see how easy it can be to take better care of the mind, body, and spirit that you've been given. Sure, it takes energy to exercise. But it always feels great. Sure, fresh ingredients may take a few seconds longer to prepare. But a well-lived life is one that is well worth living! And now it's easier than ever to begin.

In fact, to launch yourself into loving a fitter new you, simply follow along as the 21-Day Jamba Juice Lifestyle Plan unfolds. Soon you will see how easy it is to start at a low level and slowly build up. You will realize how revitalizing drinking a fresh fruit smoothie each day can be. In fact, if your short-term goal is enhanced health and a decreased risk for numerous diseases, getting into the swing of forty to sixty minutes of exercise five days a week can work miracles. In my practice, I've seen it happen time and time again. Already wondering if you can find the time?! Get creative. Think outside the box. If you want to watch TV after work, simply exercise at the same time, and imagine how fit you will soon be.

What's even better is that Kirk is not asking you to become a body builder who spends hours every day flexing in front of a mirror. His plan gently guides you toward finding activities that *you* consider fun! This is a plan that will work! Kirk Perron has put together a fun and simple plan for you that involves colorfully good nutrition, from reliable resources such as the American Heart Association, The National Institutes of Health, and the American Cancer Society—just to name a few. He has gathered together dozens of delicious, healthful, easy-to-make smoothie and juice recipes. He has mapped out a program designed to boost your metabolism and increase your emotional well-being.

I encourage you to enjoy every savory morsel of this book, have fun with it, and remember that you are worth the attention you devote to yourself. Those loving people you are surrounded by are worth it too. Don't they deserve to be with you for a long, long time?

—LEE LIPSENTHAL, M.D.
Medical Director, Lifestyle Advantage and the Dr. Dean
    Ornish Program for Reversing Heart Disease
Vice President and President-Elect, the American Board
    of Holistic Medicine

Introduction

It's hard for me to believe but when I opened my first juice and smoothie store in San Luis Obispo, California, in 1990 I naturally hoped it would be a success, but I never would have dreamed then that in just a few short years there would be over 350 Jamba Juice stores across the country, let alone that I'd be written about in the *New York Times* and the *Wall Street Journal* or that I would appear on *Oprah* or be named one of San Francisco's fifty most powerful people. I was a small-town boy who never graduated from college. But that's exactly what happened.

But this book isn't meant to be a business success story. It's simply meant to help you bring the essence of our uplifting, nutritionally packed, fruit-filled Jamba Juice experience home with you, while providing the additional key ingredients needed for a healthier lifestyle—including information on balancing the other food groups, interesting movement and

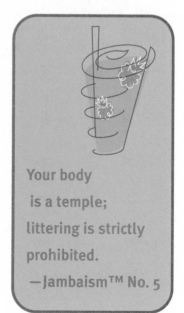

Your body
is a temple;
littering is strictly
prohibited.
—Jambaism™ No. 5

stress reduction ideas, how to become more positive, and my simple step-by-step 21-Day Smoothie and Juice Guide.

Why did I decide to write a book? I know from my own experience and from talking to customers that we have all become multitaskers on the run. It's hectic out there! We need practical ways to keep our energy levels up, our bodies in shape, and our brains functioning at maximum capacity. Yet, because we are so busy, we don't always eat the right foods or treat our bodies the way we should, which only adds to our fatigue and stress levels. I know there are hundreds of books on diet and nutrition on the market, books that sometimes contradict one another or provide complicated plans that are impossible to maintain—not to mention the ones that are questionable in their healthiness factor. Of course,

I won't be suggesting that you eat *pork rinds for breakfast*! Seriously, though, I know from talking to our customers that they are often confused by all the information they are bombarded with. I know that what people really want is to feel more confident about their lifestyle choices without stressing out over exact equations or counting calories or food exchanges 24/7.

That's why I decided to write a book that does exactly what Jamba Juice does—approaches the topic of health and diet in a simple, easy-to-understand way in the context of twenty-one days of smoothies, simple nutritional alternatives, and fun physical activities that anyone can make a part of their daily life. And it's all based on what Jamba Juice does best—unleashing the power of vitamin-packed fruit smoothies and juices.

Over the years I've heard from hundreds of people that Jamba Juice is often their first introduction to healthier eating, but it's also reflective of an entire lifestyle. Eating a little better and moving our bodies a little more not only makes us look great and feel good—it can be a whole lot of fun!

So for years it has been my mission and passion to get the word out on how easy it can be to live a more vibrant lifestyle just by making a few simple yet healthier choices in what you eat and do with your body. And as you are about to find out, the same philosophy and energy that built Jamba Juice into a phenomenon has been poured into this book.

In fact, my philosophy in life and for Jamba Juice has always been to maintain integrity, maintain balance, have self-respect, believe in yourself, and have fun. It's a holistic mind/body approach to good health. My belief is that if I can get one person on the road to eating healthy, I've also helped him or her get on the road to an overall sense of well-being. It has become my mission, not just through the growth and consistency of our stores but through my work in Jamba Juice–sponsored charities, fund-raisers, and community events, as well as through my public speaking, to get the word out on the importance of achieving a healthier lifestyle without being intimidating or preachy. I want to provide the pleasure, good nutrition, and message of an active lifestyle that Jamba Juice has come to stand for and let you, the reader, bring it home with you.

A Brief History of Jamba®

In 1990, I was a twenty-six-year-old fitness buff living in San Luis Obispo, California. After long bike rides or intense workouts at the gym I wanted something to replenish my body and mind—something quick and convenient—but I couldn't stomach grabbing a bag of chips and a candy bar, or going to another fast-food joint for a greasy cheeseburger, fatty fries, and a supersized soda. So one day, after a particularly long bike ride, I treated myself to a smoothie at the local granola and grunge health-food stand and something inside of me clicked. Maybe people would stop relying on empty-calorie foods if someone created a life-nourishing, affordable, convenient alternative.

I realized then and there that freshly made smoothies and juices were the ticket. You can enjoy smoothies on the run, they taste fantastic, they don't cost a lot, and their health benefits are undeniable. I studied the market a little further, found a location near the Cal Poly campus that would attract customers I felt would enjoy smoothies the most, bought a few industrial-strength blenders, and gathered the best possible fruits and vegetables I could find. Along with a core group of passionate like-minded individuals, within one year of my entrepreneurial epiphany, the "Juice Club®" was born.

Despite a somewhat disappointing summer (most of the college kids go home during the break, whoops!), Juice Club became a success soon thereafter. Not to brag, but our smoothies and fresh squeezed juices tasted better than anything on the market, and our atmosphere was fun, hip, and young. That first store was a spot where customers could finally gather and feel good about what they were putting into their bodies.

By late fall, our energetic atmosphere and freshly blended smoothies and juices began attracting runners, bikers, and triathletes, as well as vegetarians, vegans, and organic eaters. Within a few more months, I noticed that active teens, skateboarders, soccer players, and surfers were surging in for an afternoon pick-me-up. As word of mouth spread, I noticed more and more health-conscious hipsters and high-powered movers and shakers coming in for early-morning energy boosts. Seniors started strolling in to indulge in guilt-free, rejuvenating evening snacks. And parents trying to find a nutritious snack for themselves as well as one that their kids would enjoy began coming in at all hours of the day. My first store became a certifiable small-town hit.

Before long Juice Club's growth reflected the demand of our loyal and enthusiastic customers. Along with the help of franchising by the third anniversary, our dedicated team—consisting of only Kevin Peters, Joe Vergara, Linda Ozawa, and myself—managed to open our second store. Slowly and surely everything was falling into place until we realized that to expand, without compromising our standards, we needed to operate our own stores. Enter: Venture Financing—which would help us grow more consistently and efficiently by selling stock in the company to venture capitalists. That's when we brought in a few of the best and brightest heavy hitters in the league of big business: savvy leaders and other top-notch venture capitalists who became our first board of directors.

After the business pros came on board, a decision was quickly made to capture the essence of Juice Club and redefine it with a new name that would better embody the experience that kept customers coming back day after day. The African word *jama* was discovered, which means "to celebrate," and that helped me come up with our brand's new distinctive name, Jamba Juice.

For the next few years everything fell smoothly into place . . . and while Juice Club is still an important brand of the company, changing the name to Jamba Juice and reorganizing our priorities helped us begin growing like a weed. In fact, people flocked into our stores at an amazing pace. Reporters were calling asking for interviews, Deans of colleges were asking me to give speeches, and I even got to appear as a guest on the Queen of Daytime TV's *Oprah*. Life was good. So much so, that at one point in 1998, we were opening two stores a week for months on end—that's pretty incredible.

Jamba Juice has become a West Coast phenomenon that is sweeping the country with stores in just about every major

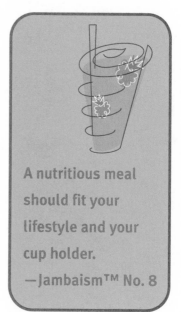

A nutritious meal should fit your lifestyle and your cup holder.

—Jambaism™ No. 8

market. In addition to over 350 stores, Jamba can be found in-side twenty-five Whole Foods Markets, fifteen universities, and three major airports, and I hope to see it expand into hundreds more stores within the next few years.

Today, the Jamba Juice brand is celebrated for its quality, its natural ingredients, and its nutritional know-how and benefits. And we continue to keep everything as natural and unspoiled as we can.

More than just healthful smoothies, Jamba Juice represents an attitude about healthy living that resonates clearly with its ever-growing audience. We also believe each food choice we make has a major impact on our personal well-being and the health of our communities—our entire planet, for that matter—so we have committed ourselves to continuing to make healthier living quick, delicious, and fun.

So what do we do that is getting millions of people excited? We sell good health and nutrition, in a cup—a playful lifestyle in a freshly blended smoothie! For the full Jamba experience, visit your local Jamba Juice store.

Now I want to make it easier for you to have the same bene-fits of Jamba when you can't make it into one of our stores.

Chapter 1

Why Fruit?

Fruit is the ultimate gift from Mother Nature. We are reminded of this every time we serve a smoothie in our store. Naturally sweet and often sensually juicy, fruit not only tickles your taste buds, but it's packed with essential vitamins, minerals, fiber, and other helpful nutrients. Fruits are also extremely versatile. You can bake fruit into pies, dry it into snacks, or add fruit to whole-grain cereals, rice, casseroles and many other tantalizing entrees. And you can freeze fruit for later use or blend different fruits into smoothies and go-go-go!

Fantastic fruits (and potent vegetables) are naturally low in fat and excellent sources of vitamins A, C, E, B_6, beta-carotene, folic acid, and selenium—to name just a few. Plus, fruits contain powerful amounts of antioxidants and phytochemicals—those extraordinary, free-radical–fighting agents—that can help your body in the battle against all sorts of

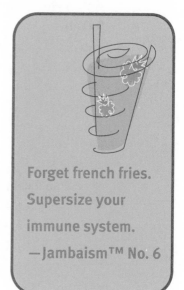

Forget french fries. Supersize your immune system.
—Jambaism™ No. 6

things like the signs of aging and other ailments such as cancer and heart disease.

What *exactly* are antioxidants, phytochemicals, and free radicals? you ask.

✳ **Antioxidants** can help defend your body against free radicals or unstable molecules that can destroy healthy cells through a process called oxidation, the same process that turns the inside of many fruits brown after you cut into them. Antioxidants are like little soldiers acting as your body's first line of defense to fight off as many free-radical rebels as they possibly can. Antioxidants come in the form of vitamins (A, C, E, beta-carotene), minerals such as selenium, and phytochemicals. Sometimes when they are strong enough they can repair free-radical damage, which can mean you will look younger for a lot longer!

✳ **Free radicals** are basically unstable oxygen molecules in your body that are produced any time your body transforms food into energy and even as often as when you breathe in and out. You also experience external free radical exposure from things like sunlight (UV light), X rays, smoking, alcohol, heat, and some forms of pollution. Free radicals can cause serious cell damage that doctors have recently linked to many age related diseases, including arthritis and osteoporosis (bone weakening), as well as to heart disease and stroke.

✳ **Phytochemicals,** or **phytonutrients,** are similar to antioxidants. In fact, some phytochemicals are powerful antioxidants and come in the form of retinoids, carotenoids, and other plant components. Put simply, *phyto* is derived from a Greek word meaning plant. Phytonutrients are made up of compounds that give fruits and vegetables their distinctive colors (retinoids and carotenoids), sensuous aromas, and intoxicating flavors.

These compounds are called pigments and flavonoids. Research shows that they can help slow down all sorts of diseases and health problems, especially those associated with aging. Plus, new scientific evidence suggests that phytonutrients found in fruits and veggies can help strengthen your immune system, eliminate cancer cells, and repair damage caused by things like cigarette smoke (even secondhand). Of course, I am not giving you permission to light up. In fact, for your health's sake make a date to stop smoking and just do it!

Sound a bit overwhelming? Relax and think of it this way: *Oxidation* is simply the process that turns an apple brown soon after you slice into it. But if you had drenched the apple in lemon juice right after slicing into it, the vitamin C in the lemon juice—a powerful *antioxidant*—you would have stopped the browning process. Just like the apple, antioxidants inside your body can stop free radicals before they can do any damage to your cells. In doing so, they can help prevent a bunch of serious diseases from coming your way.

So, just by eating plenty of fruits (and vegetables) each day, along with a balanced diet, you can supply your body with many of the important antioxidants and phytochemicals it needs to keep you looking young and feeling superstrong.

So how do you best take advantage of fruit?

We've all heard that certain fruits are good for certain things. Maybe you mentally link oranges with vitamin C or bananas with potassium. But the truth is that every fruit (and vegetable) is a multidimensional disease fighter. For instance, one glass of OJ contains 170 different phytochemicals—plus other beneficial ingredients like thiamin, folate, potassium, as well as a bushel of vitamin C, according to top researchers at Tufts University. Oranges and red beans and okra, which are high in folic acid, may improve your love life because folic acid helps keep arteries clear so blood can flow to the right places (wink, wink). Apples, grapefruit pulp, and carrots can help lower bad cholesterol (LDL). Other foods high in beta-carotene, like sweet potatoes, pumpkin, and spinach, may help diminish the damage caused to your system by bad cholesterol.

Is there an easy way to understand what cholesterol actually does?

Think about cholesterol as a member of the fat family—a somewhat distant cousin, if you will. In small amounts, cholesterol can do good things, like help build cell membranes, as well as build brain and nerve tissues. It also helps regulate the body and process food through digestion. What many don't realize is that your body is very efficient and makes all the cholesterol it needs, thanks mostly to your liver. In fact, adults don't need to eat *any* extra cholesterol. In reality, however, our diets are usually bogged down with all sorts of cholesterol-packed items like fatty meats, whole-milk products, and egg yolks.

Notice any similarity? Foods from animals contain the highest levels of cholesterol. And if you choose to eat too many animal-related products laden with cholesterol (and saturated fats), like butter, eggs, and whole milk, what you are basically doing is creating a mini-dam of white, waxy, bad cholesterol (LDL), which could eventually stop the blood from flowing freely through your veins and arteries. Not good.

Your Quick and Easy Guide to Good and Bad Cholesterol

Today we know that the *total* amount of cholesterol in food is not necessarily the only villain. Yes, the *oxidized cholesterol* in your blood, a transport device known as LDL (low-density lipoprotein), is a big part of the problem that may lead you down the low road to disease central. But the other part of the problem is simply the sheer volume of fat that many of us over-indulge in. Too many fats of any kind in your diet, especially saturated fats and trans-fatty acids found in processed food, lead to an increase in bad cholesterol, which, as mentioned before, causes plaque to build up inside the walls of your arteries. In a nutshell, go for less fat and more fruits and veggies!

Good cholesterol is called HDL (aka high-density lipoprotein). HDLs are cool because they travel through your blood like mini trash collectors and pick up all the used and unused cholesterol. Then they take the bad stuff back to your liver to be recycled. That's why experts from the FDA, USDA, American Dietetics Association, and the American Institute for Cancer Research tell us that people who exercise and eat plenty of

FACT FUNFASTFACT FUNFASTFACT FUNFASTFACT FUNFASTFACT
UNFASTFACT FUNFASTFACT FUNFASTFACT FUNFASTFACT FUNFA

Blood brings nutritious substances to cells and washes away the waste 24/7. Pumped by your heart, blood flows through veins, arteries, and capillaries. In your lifetime your heart will pump enough blood to fill one hundred full-sized swimming pools.

fruits and veggies and other healthy ingredients (including an optional glass of red wine a day) often have higher levels of HDLs, so they are less at risk for cardiovascular diseases because the bad gunk is cleared from their bloodstreams more often. Of course, if you eat nutritiously and exercise regularly you have less junk to get rid of in the first place and therefore your HDL levels may actually be lower. As always, check with your doctor to make sure your cholesterol levels are healthy for *you*.

Now you know a little about the powerful benefits of fruit. Remember, the best way to take advantage of fruit's amazing properties is to choose to eat a minimum of two to four servings of fruits every day. Luckily, all the smoothies that I will teach you to make may help provide you with many of the nutrients your body needs to look and feel good. The other thing to remember before beginning my twenty-one-day guide is to not limit yourself to eating *only* apples or eating *only* oranges. Just like humans each fruit has its own list of unique and beneficial properties. So if you want to get the biggest bang for your nutritional buck, the USDA recommends you eat a balanced diet that includes an international variety of colorful fruits (and veggies) every day so you can maximize their different benefits. Great health is all about choices. If you want it, keep those colorful fruits and vegetables coming!

Why Smoothies?

Smoothies along with balanced meals and daily exercise can help you look and feel stronger, slimmer, sexier, and healthier. Smoothies are a fantastic alternative for sweet-tooth cravings, they're easy to make, and can be eaten on the run. Smoothies make good snacks because they fill you up and may provide you with a long-lasting energy boost—all without any caffeine. They can be added to, or substituted for, breakfast, lunch, or dinner if you like. In other words, smoothies are the ultimate fast food!

Because smoothies can fill you up quickly and may help give you energy for hours, they can also be used as sensible light meal replacements, especially when you begin striving toward eating five to six smaller meals, which helps boost metabolism and burn calories. Consider for example that each of the five to six smaller meals in an average 2,000-calorie-a-day diet would be about 400 calories of varying nutritional benefit. Most of our twenty-four-ounce fruit smoothies range from 400 to 450 calories and are packed with vitamins, minerals, fiber, and phytonutrients, and each of our 24- to 32-ounce fruit smoothies contains three to five servings of fruit, nonfat yo-gurt, ice or sherbet.

In case you're confused about the bat-tle between good carbs versus bad carbs,

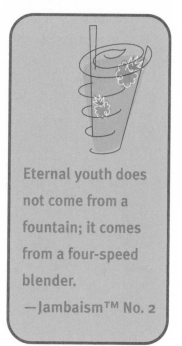

Eternal youth does not come from a fountain; it comes from a four-speed blender.

—Jambaism™ No. 2

the carbohydrates found in smoothies are the good ones, both simple and complex (which we'll discuss further in a few pages). And despite the high-protein diet craze, your body does 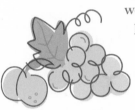 need carbs. In fact, for active people of normal weight your body and brain need plenty of carbs! How many? Leading health authorities, such as WHO (World Health Organization), ADA (American Dietetic Association), and the USDA, recommend a carbohydrate intake of 55 to 70 percent of calories consumed, which works out to about 1,100 to 1,400 daily carbohydrate calories or 275 to 350 grams a day.

Of course, please note that many people, especially women trying to maintain or lose weight, may not need more than 1,200 to 1,500 calories per day in order to maintain their weight, partly because they may be inactive. The good news is that in either case, most of the smoothies I'm about to teach you how to make, as well as the ones sold in our stores, contain an average of 100 grams of carbs, which is about 400 calories. So you get a third of the carbohydrates you need each day— both complex and simple—all from Mother Nature's medicine chest of nutrient-rich fruits.

Why 21 Days?

Behavior science tells us that it takes twenty-one days to change a bad habit into a good one, reports the American Academy of Family Physicians. For example, twenty-one days after you quit smoking it's likely you have found other things to occupy your time and energy, so for the most part your cravings have stopped. You now call yourself a nonsmoker. Or, let's say you start an exercise program. When you stick with it for twenty-one days, it becomes routine, more likely to be a reality of your everyday life. After twenty-one days you naturally begin to say things like, "Oh, I am a power walker." Or, "I do yoga to stay in shape." Or, "My arms? . . . Oh, I lift weights."

In essence I have taken that same idea and simply expanded on it. I have mapped out each day for you to include one healthful smoothie idea, tips on incorporating healthier food choices into your life, as well as some easy ways for you to become more active. After the twenty-one days are over you will have tried about twenty-one new smoothie recipes, and you will have seen how easy it can be to incorporate almost 100 unique new foods and activities into your daily life that may just help your mind, body, and spirit rise to new heights!

The world of health and nutrition is an ongoing science often filled with complicated equations, weird-looking medical words, long-winded sentences, and endless streams of studies that beget more studies. It's confusing! That is why I've taken out as much of the scientific-sounding medical mumbo-jumbo as I possibly could, so that each step in my twenty-one-day fruit-filled guide is very simple. You will not be asked to follow complicated food combinations or calculate numerical figures from complex equations. You will not be forced to do any calorie counting or listen to any drill-sergeant-like exercise instructions from some know-it-all nerd. Case closed.

After all, most of us go on and off diet and exercise programs faster than a carousel goes around. Each time we start a new one we think, "This will be the one that changes the way I eat" or "This will make me lose all the weight I want." A few days later, we lose interest and give up. The diet didn't work! But what are we really doing when we seek a magic-bullet cure or we try to follow a strange new diet that eliminates whole food groups? We are setting ourselves up for failure.

My guide is different because I want you to win. I want to give you more tools to make more confident choices. I want to help you to make minor, healthier changes that last a lifetime. Most important, I want you to have fun along the way—and continue having fun into your youthful old age. At your own pace.

This guide isn't about deprivation; it's about adding pleasure to your life and feeling good. Again, it doesn't have a temporary lose-ten-pounds-in-two-weeks-only-to-regain-it-when-you-stop mentality. Weight loss may be a side effect, more energy may be a side effect, an improved mood may be a side effect, but ultimately it's about taking good care of yourself and feeding your body the five to nine servings of fruits and vegetables the National Cancer Institute recommends you need in order for it to function optimally.

Each fruitful day of the 21-Day Guide includes substituting one nutrient-packed smoothie for some less healthy dietary habit, a few more simple yet healthy eating ideas, at least one way to add a few minutes of physical movement to your life, and a fresh tip on how to achieve and maintain more mental balance. These twenty-one days will go by quickly. Almost effortlessly your mind may feel refreshed, your body may become a little more toned, and your spirit may feel more uplifted. Ultimately, however, it's about having fun while taking care of number one: you.

Chapter 2

Power Foods, Power Fruits, and Jamba Boosts™!

Variety might be the spice of life but when it comes to nutrition, variety is the spicy king of awesome health. In fact, choosing to eat a zesty array of power foods can boost your chances of achieving radiant skin, a sexier silhouette, increased energy, eyes that sparkle, and a razor-sharp mind—just to name a few benefits. So what exactly do I mean by power foods, power fruits, and Jamba Boosts?

Power Foods

Each day your body needs a good balance of what I like to call *power foods*, which the medical community is more likely to call carbohydrates, proteins, fats, and wa-

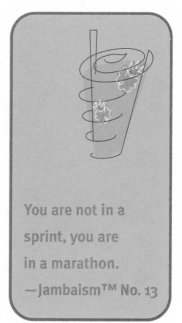

You are not in a sprint, you are in a marathon.
—Jambaism™ No. 13

ter. In fact, in an average diet of 2,000 calories a day, the World Health Organization, USDA, and other authorities recommend that about 300 grams come from carbohydrates, 50 grams from proteins, and less than 20 grams from saturated fats. If you prefer percentages, strive for 55 to 60 percent of calories to come from carbs, 10 to 20 percent from proteins, and 20 to 30 percent from fats. Oh, and drink plenty of fluids, including plain water, which many experts believe means about eight 8-ounce glasses a day.

Within that balance of power foods your body needs a certain number of vitamins, minerals, and other key nutrients to prevent nutrient deficiencies. For almost fifty years Americans relied on a complicated set of guidelines called RDAs (Recommended Daily Allowances) to help us achieve that balance. Today's standard, called RDIs (Reference Daily Intakes), is very similar in values but a lot easier to follow. Take a look at the following general guide of RDIs:

Nutrients	Based on a 2,000-calorie daily intake
Total Fat	less than 65 grams
Saturated Fat	less than 20 grams
Cholesterol	less than 300 milligrams
Sodium	less than 2,400 milligrams
Potassium	3,500 milligrams
Total Carbohydrates	300 grams
Sugars	no RDI limit set (the USDA recommends 40 grams of refined sugar or less)
Dietary Fiber	25 grams
Protein	50 grams
Vitamin A	5,000 I.U. (International Units)
Beta-Carotene	5 milligrams
Vitamin C	60 milligrams
Calcium	1,000 milligrams

Iron	18 milligrams
Vitamin E	30 I.U.
Phosphorus	1,000 milligrams
Thiamin B_1	1.5 milligrams
Riboflavin B_2	1.7 milligrams
Niacin B_3	20 milligrams
Vitamin B_6	2.0 milligrams
Vitamin B_{12}	6 micrograms
Folic Acid	400 micrograms
Vitamin D	400 I.U.
Vitamin K	80 micrograms
Biotin	300 micrograms
Pantothenic Acid	10 milligrams
Magnesium	400 milligrams
Zinc	15 milligrams
Copper	2 milligrams
Manganese	2 milligrams
Selenium	70 micrograms
Chloride	3,400 milligrams
Iodine	150 micrograms
Molybdenum	75 micrograms
Chromium	120 micrograms

RDI, "Reference Daily Intakes," comprise of a set of reference values for specific nutrients, each category of which has special usages. This comprehensive effort to establish RDIs is headed by the Scientific Evaluation of Daily Reference Intakes of Food and Nutrition Board, Institute of Medicine, the National Academies, in collaboration with Health Canada. The table can be referenced to FDA's Code of Federal Regulations, Title 21, Volume 2, Part 101, Section 101.9 (2002).

Please note that the world of vitamins, minerals, and supplements is ever changing. Each day scientists make new discoveries, researchers divulge the results of new studies, and doctors find new cures. For now, these RDIs are accepted as an overall general guide to the amount of vitamins and minerals that the average healthy person should be consuming from food to prevent nutrient deficiencies. However, these same RDIs are also currently being reevaluated to see if they are in amounts high enough to prevent deficiencies *and* prevent disease.

Power Fruits

At Jamba, we are constantly searching for more natural ways to maximize our customers' nutritional needs. I coined the term *power fruits* to simply describe for you some of the most powerful fruits on the planet, the whole gamut of which are blended into millions of Jamba smoothies every year. What's so great about power fruits? Power fruits may help you get one step closer to achieving your nutritional goals because they are packed with essential vitamins, minerals, amino acids, and certain fatty acids.

Jamba Boosts™

Even if you eat a balanced diet it may be tough to get all the generally recommended amounts of nutrients you need. Plus, if you have special dietary needs you may need *more* nutrients. For instance, maybe your body is lacking certain nutrients because you are under a lot of stress, or trying to safely lose weight, or

FACT FUNFASTFACT FUNFASTFACT FUNFASTFACT FUNFASTFACT
UNFASTFACT FUNFASTFACT FUNFASTFACT FUNFASTFACT FUNFA

Did you know that it's estimated up to 70 percent of all Americans and nearly 60 percent of our medical doctors take supplements? That's because vitamin and mineral supplements taken regularly can help fill in the possible gaps in an imperfect diet.

have a family history of heart disease. That's where Jamba Boosts can help. Basically, our boosts are high quality, effective supplements designed to help boost your body and mind, some on a daily basis to ensure you are getting the adequate number of RDIs and some for those few days when you may need an extra boost, perhaps during cold and flu season. All of our boosts can be added into any of our smoothie recipes. Of course, we call them boosts, but some members of the health and science community would also call them *nutraceuticals*.

Okay, now that you have a brief and general understanding of all three categories let's start exploring exactly how power foods, power fruits, and Jamba Boosts may help you!

Power Foods

Power foods are the first and most important ingredients needed for life: water, carbohydrates, proteins, and fats. Let's take a look at why.

Water

Your body is almost two-thirds water. Water is used to help perform every function in your body. Without water your body could not carry nutrients from one place to the next, nor could you eliminate waste. Water is vital to life. It helps your body temperature remain constant. Water helps lubricate your joints so you can continue bending, lifting your arms and walking. And to ensure great health choose to drink approximately eight 8-ounce glasses of water every day.

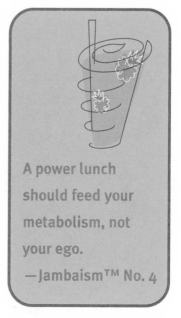

A power lunch should feed your metabolism, not your ego.

—Jambaism™ No. 4

Carbohydrates

Carbohydrates give your body and mind the energy you need to function. The best carbs are found naturally in fruits, vegetables, whole grains, legumes, peas, and beans. You can also get carbohydrates from milk and milk products. You've probably heard the terms *simple carbs* and *complex carbs*. They are simply the two main groups carbohydrates are divided into.

✳ **Simple carbs** are often referred to as simple sugars and include things like whole fruits, fruit sugar (or fructose), table sugar (sucrose), and milk sugar (lactose), as well as a few lesser-known ones.

✳ **Complex carbs** are made up of sugars too. But they are strung together to form longer, much more complex chains. Complex carbs include fiber and starches. Foods full of complex carbs include whole fruits, vegetables, whole grains, peas, and beans.

Your body needs both kinds of carbohydrates because they are converted by your body into something called *blood glucose,* which is the most important fuel for cells and the only real source of energy for your brain and red blood cells. Your body either uses the glucose for energy or stores it for later in the form of fat.

It's best to eat plenty of complex carbs as mentioned above and avoid too many simple, more refined carbs found in processed foods like soda, candy, and many desserts. Why? Besides helping to cause weight gain, an excess of simple carbs can lead to many health problems, especially diabetes (a disorder where the body can't make proper use of carbohydrates) and hypoglycemia (low blood sugar) and tooth decay.

Fiber, or roughage as many of us know it, is an important complex carb that benefits us in many ways. As discussed already, because most fiber is not actually digested it pushes things through our systems in the form of proper waste management. Fiber helps prevent constipation and hemorrhoids. When you choose a high-fiber diet your chances of colon cancer are greatly diminished. Fiber also helps lower your levels of bad cholesterol (LDL).

Protein

You need protein for growth. Protein also helps provide your body with energy. You need protein so your body can produce growth hormones, enzymes, and antibodies to help fight infections and illness. Plant proteins from things like beans and nuts, as well as animal proteins found in meat, poultry, and fish, help provide the essential amino acids you need for good health.

Fats

Your body needs fats to survive, especially the "good" fats found in things like fish, olive oil, and flaxseeds. Fat provides energy, structural integrity of cells and membranes, and insulation—to name just a few. Because your body doesn't make its own fat or synthesize essential fatty acids, you need to get fats from your diet. Fat also acts as a carrier for the fat-soluble vitamins A, D, E, and K, and as an aid to their absorption in the intestine.

Too much fat, especially saturated fat and trans-fatty acids (formed by the process of hydrogenation to increase a product's shelf life), is a fact of life and unfortunately contributes to obesity, coronary heart disease, and other health problems. The American Heart Association recommends that you limit total fat to 30 percent of your total caloric intake and that less than 20 grams of the total be saturated fats.

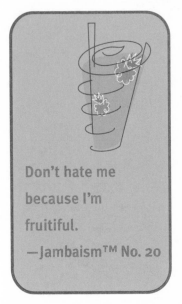

Don't hate me
because I'm
fruitiful.

—Jambaism™ No. 20

Power Fruits

In the previous chapter, you learned how valuable fruits and therefore smoothies may be in the fight against things like aging and disease because they are filled with vitamins, minerals, fiber, and powerful antioxidants. Fruits are so good for you that leading health authorities such as the National Cancer Institute, the USDA, and the American Dietetic Association all recommend five to nine servings of fruits and vegetables in your diet each day for optimal long-term health. Unfortunately, less than three out of ten people eat the recommended serving of fruits and vegetables per day, according to the Centers for Disease Control. That's why I want to point you toward the cream of the crop so power fruits may begin to work their magic on you as soon as possible.

Top Power Fruits

* **Blueberries,** *Eating Well* magazine's 1998 Fruit of the Year, are bursting with antioxidants that help protect your brain from free radicals. Plus, blueberries are packed with vitamin C to help you fight the common cold and beat stress. The vitamin A and beta-carotene in blueberries may help you prevent infections, heart disease, cancer, and strengthen immunity. Blueberries can also act as an antibiotic to help curb urinary tract infections

* **Oranges** are a powerhouse of vitamin C, one of your body's strongest antioxidants, which may help boost your immunity and absorb iron from food. Oranges also have lots of

disease-banishing compounds, including *flavonoids,* the compounds that give fruits and vegetables their bright colors, to protect your heart, fight cancer, and stomp out infections. Oranges also have the fiber pectin in them, which may help reduce bad cholesterol. And they are bursting with potassium, which may help lower blood pressure.

✳ **Strawberries.** According to researchers at Tufts University, one cup of strawberries contains 140 percent of your daily vitamin C, lots of fiber for healthy digestion, and other beneficial phytochemicals best known for their antiviral, anticancer activity. Did you also know that strawberries date back to Ancient Rome and that in the thirteenth century they were used as medicinal herbs?

✳ **Raspberries** are tops in antioxidants, including 50 percent more cancer-fighting properties than strawberries and double the fiber. Plus, one cup of raspberries is drenched with 52 percent of your daily C. And did you know that red raspberries are often called caneberries because they grow on erect stalks or canes?

✳ **Bananas** can soothe your upset stomach, stop diarrhea, and they can strengthen your tummy against acids and ulcers. Plus, bananas are bursting with antibiotic activity, and they contain plenty of fiber in the form of pectin, like oranges, which can help curb your appetite.

FACT FUNFASTFACT FUNFASTFACT FUNFASTFACT FUNFASTFACT
UNFASTFACT FUNFASTFACT FUNFASTFACT FUNFASTFACT FUNFA

Navel oranges get their name because their bottoms look like belly buttons or navels. Each year Jamba serves enough vitamin-packed orange juice to fill over 5 Olympic-sized swimming pools from top to bottom. Talk about diving into a pool of liquid refreshment!

✳ **Mangos.** Yes, mangos! An exotic fruit packed with beta-carotene needed for growth and smooth skin. One cup has 160 percent of your daily vitamin A, 95 percent of C, and 14 percent of B_6 that can help your body grow properly and may help keep you in a good mood! To prove they are bursting with antioxidants, just slice one open and see what happens. (Clue: A mango won't brown like an apple.)

✳ **Cranberries** are teaming with vitamin C, fiber, and the recently discovered antibiotic properties of large molecules called A-*linked condensed tannins* that have the unusual ability to keep infectious bacteria from sticking to cells lining your bladder and urinary tract that may help you prevent and fight those types of infections.

✳ **Grapefruit.** Eat half a grapefruit and you've fulfilled 70 percent of your daily C. Plus, grapefruits contain many cancer-fighting flavonoids as well as potassium, which may help keep your heart pumping properly. Grapefruits, like oranges and apples, are also full of cholesterol-lowering pectin. (Beware: Certain prescription drugs do not interact well with grapefruit, so ask your doctor if it's okay to include them in your diet.)

✳ **Kiwifruit** contains an avalanche of incredible vitamins and minerals. In fact, two medium kiwis will give you twice the amount of vitamin C of an orange. Plus, they are brimming with fiber, potassium, and magnesium for strong bones, teeth, and muscles.

✳ **Grapes.** In tests done at Tufts University, "Concord grape juice had four times the antioxidant power of other juices, including orange, tomato, and grapefruit," say authors of *The Color Code*. Grape juice is also great for keeping your heart healthy because like many fruits it helps lower cholesterol. Plus, the deep purple flavonoids that give grapes their gorgeous skin tone can also help keep your arteries sparkling clean and elastic enough to deliver more key nutrients to your brain, muscles, and other vital organs. (FYI: Concord grapes rank high on nutritional charts, as do other purple and red grapes.)

✳ **Avocados** (yes, they are a fruit) are filled with vitamins, beta-carotene, potassium, magnesium, fiber, and fat. *Fat?!* Not to worry, two-thirds of the fat is the good kind of mono-unsaturated fat that won't raise your bad cholesterol level. Of course, the other third is dense in calories, so go easy on this fruity choice, amigo.

Those are just a few of the most powerful fruits available. But you don't have to stop there . . . other fruits rich in nutrients include pineapples, apricots, cantaloupes, honeydews, watermelons, pears, plums, apples, blackberries, boysenberries, and cherries. From there, your list of colorful choices goes on and on and on . . .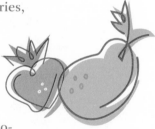

Besides choosing to drink a fruit-filled smoothie each day, here are some more instant ways to make a beautiful day like today . . . even more fruitful: Once you've topped your cereal with sliced strawberries, have a juicy green apple for a mid-morning snack. For lunch, enjoy a spinach salad topped with Mandarin orange slices. In the afternoon, have half of a cantaloupe or honeydew melon. After supper, toss a handful of blueberries on top of a petite dessert bowl filled with low-fat frozen yogurt. Tomorrow, pick a whole bunch of other fruits to appreciate. Mix it all up the day after that by starting your day with a bowl of oatmeal and kiwifruit. Have half a grapefruit after lunch with a handful of almonds. Munch on a small package of dried apricots in the afternoon. Simmer down at sunset with a bowl of ripe cherries or a handful of grapes.

Jamba Boosts™

You may have noticed that we like blending things at Jamba Juice. That's because we believe in a well-rounded approach to food and nutrition. After all, what modern-day monkey wouldn't want to drink a refreshingly cool smoothie rather than eat a pound of bananas in one sitting? So naturally when it came to creating nutritional supplements, we had to blend them too. The result: our powerful line of Jamba Boosts!

Fusing carefully chosen whole foods, herbs, and nutrients, Jamba Boosts are synergistic blends of vitamins, minerals, herbs, and botanical ingredients that may help give your body optimum support from multiple sources of important nutrients. Remember, certain amounts of daily vitamins and minerals, the RDIs, are key to a total health program. The whole topic seems complicated but it really isn't. For instance, sometimes vitamins and minerals are called *micronutrients* because your body only needs small or *micro* amounts of them, especially compared to the plentiful group I call power foods that your body needs every day such as carbs, proteins, fats, and water, which we discussed earlier.

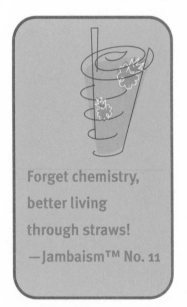

Forget chemistry, better living through straws!

—Jambaism™ No. 11

In case you're unclear as to how all these micronutrients can help or what they actually do inside your body, let me simplify. Vitamins are found naturally in many plants and animal products. Basically, vitamins function as the *companions* of enzymes, or *coenzymes*. Enzymes do all sorts of wonderful things in your body such as help you digest food and make sure the chemicals in your brain continue sending signals where needed. Without the microscopic marriage of enzymes and vitamins, you could not breathe, see, or even walk—that's how important their partnership is.

Different from vitamins but just as important, *minerals* are not found in the *organic* kingdom of plants and animals. That's why minerals are also called *inorganic elements.* Just like vitamins, minerals act as coenzymes to help your body do everything from breaking down foods that will be used for energy to connecting the nerves in your brain so that you can read this sentence.

In addition, many of our Jamba Boosts contain special herbs and botanicals. Herbs have been used in countless ways for thousands of years. Besides acting as popular sixties' song lyrics such as "Parsley, sage, rosemary and thyme" many herbs have been added to enhance the flavors of foods as well as many other unusual things. For instance, in ancient Greece, students braided rosemary into their hair to help energize their memories during exams—and they say modern kids are twisted! Anyway, today we know that many herbs are rich in protective *phyto*chemicals too. (Again, *phyto* simply means it comes from a plant.)

The word *botanical* is another term that means "derived from a plant." Many botanicals have been studied for centuries to see if they have extra medicinal powers to heal. A botanical such as ginkgo biloba comes from an ancient tree of the same name that dates back two million years! As far as we know, medicinal use of ginkgo began over five thousand years ago. This botanical has been shown to help fight fatigue, increase mental and physical stamina (including sexual), and increase your energy levels.

Now look back at the RDI chart for a moment. That's quite an overwhelming list of nutrients, isn't it? I've already pointed out a reason it's difficult to get the proper amount of RDIs of vitamins and minerals in your daily diet; others include the fact that many of us are often on the run with no time to eat balanced meals. Or we are following a strict diet, so we eat fewer calories and therefore fewer nutrients. Plus, it may be impossible to get all of the vitamins and minerals we need each day just from the food we eat because the nutrient content of many modern foods fluctuates like crazy. For instance, if a farm's soil has been overused it may have been stripped of many important minerals such as magnesium, zinc, selenium, and calcium. Therefore, fruits and vegetables grown in those poor soil conditions do not have as many nutrients as they could, or *should.*

In addition, in today's hectic world many of us may need *more* than the RDIs of vitamins and nutrients for various other reasons. Our environment has become more polluted. So we may need extra antioxidants to combat the toxins in the air we breathe or the water we drink. Some of the processed meats we choose to eat also contain cancer-causing nitrates so we may need extra vitamin C and vitamin E to protect ourselves. In addition, many of us are suffering more from mental and physical stress. What happens when you are under a lot of stress? Studies revealed by Shari Lieberman, Ph.D., in the *Real Vitamin & Mineral Book,* show that your body uses up its store of valuable vitamins and minerals a whole lot faster. That's where Jamba Boosts can come in to help.

Jamba Boosts are high-quality, effective supplements to boost your body and mind. They are essential vitamins, minerals, herbs, and botanicals all working in sync to support your new, healthier, more active lifestyle. In our stores, we use our own carefully designed boosts, based on the following criteria: We select only the highest quality vitamins, minerals, and guaranteed potency herbs for Jamba Boosts, so you get consistent quality and great nutrition every time you boost your Jamba smoothie. We take pride in carefully formulating our boosts; we aim to provide you with the best nutrition we can by basing our formulas on something called the Optimal Daily Allowance (ODA) for nutrients, which is often much higher than the standard RDIs, which we consider may not be high enough for today's growing nutritional needs.

How do we determine the Optimal Daily Allowance (ODA) for nutrients? We constantly track the latest research and make sure we know what amount of vitamins and minerals has a greater chance of enhancing and possibly improving your health. Again, the RDIs are the estimated average requirement amounts of nutrients set by the government. By providing you with the ODA of nutrients in some of our Jamba Boosts, we are simply giving you the option to add even more vitamins, minerals, botanicals, and herbs into your nutritional repertoire.

Naturally, we are careful not to exceed what we believe to be the Optimal Daily Allowance (ODA) for nutrients. We do not believe in *megadosing,* intentionally exceeding recommended ODA levels of nutrients. In fact, scientists are currently in the process of determining the safest upper levels of nutrients to prevent the possibility of future megadosing, or causing a disease of excess vitamin supplementation.

What's behind the power of specific Jamba Boosts™?

Juice Boosts can help take the guesswork out of supplementing your diet by addressing specific nutritional needs. For example, on a daily basis our Vita Boost™ formula of essential vitamins and minerals can help you get all of your vitamins and mineral needs met in one refreshing smoothie. During cold and flu season or bouts of stress, our Immunity Boost™ may help strengthen your immune system. In fact, we believe our multi-ingredient formulations are superior to single supplements for several reasons:

* Multi-ingredient formulations are designed to work in synergy together to provide you with a health solution and a targeted nutritional function.
* Plus, many people (almost 30 percent of the population) are deemed *nonresponders* to certain drugs and nutraceuticals, and *responders* to others. Therefore, your doctor may try various remedies to find one that works best for you. That's why we use two types of ginseng in our Energy Boost, for example, because your body may respond to one and not the other. In other words, many of our boosts are designed to be multifaceted to ensure the maximum chance of success.
* The body's needs are quite complex and require support from various sources. That's why you always hear about the importance of eating a balanced diet, because the body needs different forms of the same nutrition. The Jamba Boost approach is similar to this: multiple ingredients all supporting a desired function for the optimal result.

Again, your body needs all of the essential vitamins and minerals on a daily basis, outlined in the RDI table (see page 18–19), to function properly. Unfortunately, many of us are not getting all of them from the foods we are eating. To help fill in any nutritional gaps in your diet, therefore, it's considered wise by many leading authorities to supplement your nutritional needs by taking a multivitamin every single day.

Following is a list of our Jamba Boosts that are currently available in stores nationwide, with a brief description of why they may be effective for you. After each boost is an explanation about the powerful ingredients inside with a list of other supplements reported to have similar effects that you can buy and that may help you achieve the same benefits. As always, consult your doctor before beginning any new diet or fitness program.

Jamba Juice® Energy Boost™ = Mind and Body Energy

Our Jamba Juice Energy Boost may help you revitalize your energy levels with over 100 percent of your RDI of five B vitamins needed for energy and other key nutrients that may help support mental functions, improve concentration, and ensure brain cell maintenance. This boost also combines the ancient energizing Asian herbs known as ginseng and ginkgo biloba. Specifically, our formula features two of what we consider the most well-researched ginsengs, Korean and Siberian, thought to increase energy, enhance physical and mental endurance, and fight fatigue. Ginkgo biloba has been added to help increase the delivery of energy and oxygen to working cells, which may help boost your energy and brain power!

Jamba Juice Energy Boost Ingredients Per Serving†
(Serving size: 1 teaspoon)

Nutrient	Amount	Unit	%DV
Vitamin B_1 (as thiamin mononitrate)	40	mg	2,667
Vitamin B_3 (as niacinamide)	50	mg	250
Vitamin B_6 (as pyridoxine HCl)	25	mg	1,250
Vitamin B_{12} (as cyanocobalamin)	7	mcg	117
Vitamin B_5 (as D-calcium pantothenate)	150	mg	1,500
0.8% eleutherosides, 0.8mg Siberian ginseng (root, *Siberian ginseng*)	100	mg	*
0.8% eleutherosides, 0.8mg Korean ginseng (root, *Panax ginseng*)	50	mg	*
14% ginsenosides, 7mg Ginkgo biloba (leaf)	40	mg	*

Nutrient	Amount	Unit	%DV
24% ginkgo flavonglycosides, 9.6mg			
6% terpene lactones, 2.4mg			
Stevia extract (leaf)	30	mg	*
80–85% steviosides, 24–26mg			

*Daily value not established.
†Inactive ingredients: oat fiber (as filler) and calcium silicate (anticaking agent).

More About Energy-Boosting Supplements

* **Korean ginseng** (also called Panax) and **Siberian ginseng extract.** These ancient botanicals are scientifically classified as *adaptogens,* which may help the body *adapt to,* and protect itself against, the side effects of physical, chemical, and biological stress. Korean ginseng has been shown to increase athletic performance, help fight fatigue, and support immune function. Siberian ginseng is considered a safe energy stimulant and helps lessen the signs of fatigue. We use two types of ginseng because some people react best to one or the other, or both. You can usually find ginseng in capsule form or as a liquid.

* **Ginkgo biloba** is an ancient herb that increases blood flow to the brain and the rest of the body. It has been shown to help you think more clearly and sharply. It can also help fight depression and vertigo.

* **Vitamins B_1, B_3, B_5, B_6,** and **B_{12}** are very important because your cells use these B vitamins to enhance energy production, carbohydrate metabolism and nerve cell function. B vitamins also help with the manufacture of adrenal hormones and red blood cells, and support detoxification processes and a healthy immune system. Specifically: B_3, niacin, can help alleviate painful menstruation. B_6, folic acid, is necessary for the formation of your brain's neuro-

transmitters, needed for mental acuity. B_5, pantothenic acid, is necessary for energy production and the reduction of cholesterol and blood triglyceride levels.

* **Stevia extract** is used around the world as a no-calorie sweetener; the leaves of the stevia plant have a refreshing taste that can be thirty times sweeter than sugar. It can be found in powder and liquid form. In a smoothie, its pleasing sweet flavor can help mask some of the less pleasant flavors of supplements such as a powdered protein.

Jamba® Femme Boost™ = Powerful Female Nutrition

Our Jamba Femme Boost has been carefully designed for the specific daily and long-term health concerns of women, such as strong bones, healthy skin, and a comfortable menstrual cycle and menopause. Incorporating the key vitamins and minerals critical to women's health, as well as herbs that we consider highly renowned for their ability to balance the female body's special requirements.

Jamba Femme Boost Ingredients Per Serving†
(Serving size: 1 teaspoon)

Nutrient	Amount	Unit	%DV
Vitamin A (palmitate)	5,000	I.U.	100
Vitamin D (cholecalciferol)	440	I.U.	110
Folic acid	480	mcg	120
Calcium (as calcium carbonate)	1,000	mg	100
Iron (as iron fumerate)	11	mg	61

Nutrient	Amount	Unit	%DV
Magnesium (as magnesium oxide)	400	mg	100
Wild yam (*Dioscorea villosa*) (root)	150	mg	*
6% total saponins, 9mg			
Soy isoflavones	25	mg	*
Stevia extract	5	mg	*
>85% steviosides, >4.3mg			
Boron (as boron glycinate)	2	mg	*

*Daily value not established.
†Inactive ingredient: oat fiber.

More About Femme-Boosting Supplements

✳ **Soy** can be found in liquid and powder form. It's a great source of protein and contains other helpful nutrients too. In particular, soy is rich in *isoflavones,* which function as *phytoestrogens,* or plant-based nutrients, with properties similar to estrogen. These organic, microscopic nutrients help protect normal female reproductive health and comfort, especially during and after menopause. Soy isoflavones can also help support normal bone strength and density. And, according to the American Heart Association, soy protein used instead of animal protein can significantly lower bad cholesterol (LDL) without affecting the good cholesterol (HDL). However, also note that, although it has yet to be determined, excess soy may be harmful to women with high family risk of breast cancer and/or those who have breast cancer that is estrogen sensitive.

✳ **Calcium** is the most abundant mineral in the body, essential in supporting and maintaining strong, healthy bones. Bone is living tissue and needs a constant supply of calcium and other minerals in order to stay or become strong. FYI: Regular exercise and a healthy diet containing adequate cal-

cium helps women maintain good bone health
and may reduce their high risk of osteoporosis
later in life. Daily intake above 2,000 mg is
not likely to provide additional benefit.

✻ **Folic acid,** one of the B vitamins, is necessary for the efficient transformation of food
into actual energy. Folic acid supports healthy nervous system functioning, and is important (and often depleted) during times of stress. The B vitamins are also important for
maintenance of a healthy cardiovascular system. Folic acid
also supports a strong immune response.

✻ **Iron.** A menstruating woman may lose iron every month. It
is therefore important to provide the body with a continu-
ous supply of this essential trace mineral which helps blood
cells move oxygen from the lungs to every cell in the body.
A good supply of oxygen is necessary to maintain healthy
energy levels.

✻ **Magnesium** supports enzyme activity, especially energy production. Magnesium is an *electrolyte,* which is basically a
microscopic ion that cells need to regulate electric charges
and flow of water molecules across membranes. Magnesium helps support a healthy heartbeat, healthy blood pressure levels, and normal muscle relaxation.

✻ **Vitamin D** is necessary for the formation and maintenance
of strong, healthy bones and teeth. It also regulates the absorption and use of calcium.

Immunity Boost™ = Body Defense

Our Immunity Boost formula can help protect you from colds,
illness, and disease, especially during periods of stress or cold

and flu season. Immunity Boost incorporates special herbs like echinacea and olive leaf extract, minerals like zinc to enhance immune cell activity and health, and other antioxidants to help protect you against free radicals and promote overall cardiovascular health. To ensure our Immunity Boost is as balanced as possible, we have included two species and incorporated two forms of the echinacea plant. Echinacea may increase the production of white blood cells to help the body fight many diseases. In other words, this Jamba Immunity Boost helps give your body a potent line of defense from possible future attacks!

Immunity Boost Ingredients Per Serving[†]
(Serving size: ½ teaspoon)

Nutrient	Amount	Unit	%DV
Vitamin A (as beta-carotene)	5,000	I.U.	100
Vitamin C (ascorbic acid)	503	mg	838
Vitamin E (d-alpha-tocopheryl acetate)	30	I.U.	150
Zinc (as zinc gluconate)	15	mg	100
Olive leaf extract (leaf, *Olea europaea*)	200	mg	*
Echinacea blend (root, leaf)			*
E. purpurea, E. angustifolia	100	mg	*
4% phenolic compounds, 4mg			
Green Tea Extract (green, leaf)			
50% polyphenols, 50mg	100	mg	*
Stevia Extract (leaf)	15	mg	*
80–85% steviosides, 12–13mg			

*Daily value not established.
[†]Inactive ingredients: oat fiber (filler) and calcium silicate (anticaking agent).

More About Immunity-Boosting Supplements

✳ **Olive leaf extract** has been known to help your immune system keep diseases away—*the natural way.* How? The antibiotic, antiviral, and antifungal properties of chemicals found within the olive leaf (oleuropein, elenolic acid, and calcium elenolate) appear to stun microscopic invaders long enough for your body to kick into resistance mode to help keep you healthy. Olive leaf extract can be found in capsule form or enjoyed as a soothing tea as it has been for thousands of years to treat coughs, sore throats, or mild fevers.

✳ **Echinacea** enhances immune cell activity and is most commonly found in capsule form. Increasingly popular in Europe and North America, the herb is derived from the roots of the purple coneflower. Taken internally, it helps to fight bacterial and viral infections, boost the immune system, lower fever, and calm allergic reactions.

✳ **Green tea extract** contains the same powerful antioxidants found in green tea shown to reduce cholesterol and arteriosclerosis, promote a strong immune response, and help protect immune cells. The protective properties of green tea have been known for many centuries.

✳ **Zinc** plays a role in over three hundred enzymes in the body. The mineral zinc assists in the formation of DNA, the cell's genetic material. It is essential for cell division and growth. And zinc assists in the proper functioning of the hormone insulin and helps support overall immune function.

✳ **Vitamin E** functions primarily as an antioxidant in protecting against damage to cell membranes. It is important to general health and immune function.

✳ **Beta-carotene** is a precursor to vitamin A that helps protect the body from free radicals, and is important for a strong immune response. Its antioxidant properties protect and support the repair of immune cells and strengthen and sustain healthy mucous membranes of respiratory, digestive and urinary tracts, which are a first line of defense against the invasion of foreign substances.

* **Vitamin C** is also extremely well known for its ability to support and protect a strong immune system. This vitamin helps support the healthy production of immune cells such as *lymphocytes*; and protects immune cells through its antioxidant properties.
* **Stevia extract** has a pleasing flavor that helps mask some of the vitamin flavors.

Jamba Juice® Fiber Boost™ = Better Digestive Health

Fiber Boost promotes terrific digestive health. This boost is enhanced with *psyllium* (a well-known Eurasian botanical) to promote regularity, pectin to improve digestion and nutrient absorption, and acidophilus to promote healthy bacteria to stimulate your immune system and protect against infection.

In case you didn't know, fiber from plants is necessary for normal digestion of foods. There are two main groups of fibers, soluble and insoluble. *Soluble* fiber delays the stomach's emptying time as well as the transit of food through the small intestine—this improves digestion and absorption of nutrients. Soluble fiber also helps support healthy cholesterol levels. *Insoluble* fiber speeds up the time it takes for eaten matter to move through the large intestine, which means toxins have less time to sit in the colon. And when push comes to

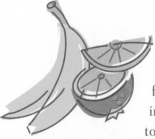

shove—pardon the pun—all this adds up to good old-fashioned regularity. That's why our Fiber Boost features a balance of more than 6 grams of fiber, both soluble and insoluble.

For those who would like to understand this subject further, soluble and insoluble fiber working together slows the breakdown of carbohydrates and delays glucose absorption into the blood, thereby supporting healthy blood sugar levels. They also provide a healthy environment for *probiotic*, a friendly bacteria; and *acidophilus*, another friendly *and* protective bacteria. So besides all the fiber, our boost has also been infused with active cultures, also known as *beneficial bacteria*, that improve vitamin absorption, protect your gastrointestinal tract from infection, and hinder the growth of disease-causing bacteria.

The specific strain of active cultures formulated into our Fiber Juice Boost is called *Lactobacillus acidophilus*; it is a friendly intestinal flora lactic bacteria culture. It is an indigenous strain (meaning they are naturally occurring and permanent in the human digestive tract) that lives in the small and large intestines. The body requires a healthy population of intestinal flora, which are critical to the proper digestion and absorption of food, the synthesis of vitamins by the body, and the maintenance of the body's immune system.

In addition, many medical studies have proven that a diet high in fiber can help lower bad cholesterol (LDL) and substantially reduce the risk of many chronic diseases including heart disease.

Jamba Juice Fiber Boost Ingredients Per Serving[†]
(Serving size: 1 tablespoon)

Nutrient	Amount	Unit	%DV
Total fiber	6.3	g	25%
Blond psyllium (seed and husk)	3.28	g	*
Oat fiber	3.5	g	*
Wheat bran	500	mg	*

Nutrient	Amount	Unit	%DV
Apple pectin (fruit)	250	mg	*
Fructooligosaccharides (FOS)	250	mg	*
Lactobacillus acidophilus	200	mg	*
1 billion organisms**			
Stevia extract (leaf)			
80–85% steviosides, 16–17mg	20	mg	*

*Daily value not established.
**At time of manufacture.
†Inactive ingredients: none.

More About Fiber-Boosting Supplements

＊ **Psyllium** is generally found in seed form and must be mixed with a liquid. It is also the active ingredient of many laxatives and can be found in some cereals. This fiber comes from the seeds of the psyllium plant, which grows in India and other parts of the Middle East. Psyllium is an excellent source of soluble fiber, which promotes regularity. It is one of the most common and well-known fiber sources.

＊ **Wheat bran** is an insoluble fiber. Bran comes from the outer hull of the seed of wheat grain. Wheat bran is one of the main reasons that whole grain wheat bread is so good for you. Generally, you can find wheat bran in its natural seed-like state or ground into a powdered form such as wheat germ. Wheat is a very popular grain that's cultivation dates back ten thousand years. Wheat can be used to create many familiar products, including breads, pastas, cereals, bulgur wheat, couscous, and wheat germ. Only buy *whole* wheat products, as the key nutrients are contained in the outer layers or husks of the wheat shaft.

＊ **Apple pectin.** Pectin is found inside many vegetables and fruits, such as grapes, apples, peaches, plums, and berries,

with its greatest abundance in citrus fruits. Pectin is derived mostly from fruits and has been commonly used in jel-
lies as a thickening agent. However, this water-soluble fiber
is now becoming known for its powerful health benefits.
Specifically, pectin is in the intercellular and cell walls of
fruits and veggies. The pectin in our Fiber Juice Boost is derived from apples. Pectin is a water-soluble fiber, which
helps slow transit time, thereby improving digestion and absorption. This complex carbohydrate may help keep your
cholesterol low. Pectin also helps protect against the toxic
effects of some of the chemicals we eat in our food. It improves glucose tolerance, does not upset electrolyte (mineral) balance, and slows gastric emptying time (rate at which
food leaves the stomach) for improved nutrient absorption.

* **Oat fiber** helps support healthy digestion, normal cholesterol levels, and a healthy cardiovascular system.

* **Fructooligosaccharides.** I dare you to *try* to say that one fast
one time. Let alone *three* times! Wow! That's why fructooligosaccharides are usually referred to simply as FOS.
FOS are naturally occurring compounds, present in many
fruits, vegetables, and grains, such as onions, asparagus roots,
tubers of Jerusalem artichokes, and wheat. FOS are non-
digestible, so they pass through the upper gastrointestinal
tract essentially intact and unabsorbed. Then they enter the
intestine, where they are available for the utilization of
friendly bacteria (probiotics), such as acidophilus.

* **L. acidophilus** is the most well known of the friendly bacteria or microorganisms (probiotics) that live in our colon
in a true symbiotic, beneficial relationship with us. These
friendly bacteria stimulate our immune system, create a
healthy environment within the colon, and form a physical
barrier to protect us against an overgrowth of bad bacteria
as well as yeast. They also support your digestive process
(including the digestion of lactose and the production of

some B vitamins), as well as colon health and function (including normal bowel movements). In fact, we cannot live without the protection of these good bacteria! Long live *L. acidophilus*!

✳ **Stevia extract** has a sweet flavor that helps masks some of the vitamin flavors.

Jamba® Multi-Boost™ = Complete Nutrition

For those searching for a daily supplement package that combines the best of all that we have, this Multi-Boost may be just right for you! In fact, Multi-Boost is considered Jamba Juice's signature formulation because we believe it helps bring almost all of your nutritional needs together. Not only does our Multi-Boost have 100 percent or more of the currently recommended amounts of twenty vitamins and minerals, but it also offers additional nutrients that may help support energy production, endurance, weight management, and a strong immune response, plus fiber and other nutrients necessary to support the entire digestive system. Featured as part of our Jamba Powerboost smoothie, it embodies the spirit of what we consider complete nutrition with its ODA combination of vitamins, minerals, protein, fiber, antioxidants, phytonutrients, and energizing herbs. In other words, this boost can help *power* your mind and body, and therefore your spirit!

Jamba Multi-Boost Ingredients Per Serving[†]
(Serving size: 1 tablespoon)

Nutrient	Amount	Unit	%DV
Vitamin A (as retinyl palmitate)	5,000	I.U.	100
Vitamin C (as ascorbic acid)	66	mg	110

Nutrient	Amount	Unit	%DV
Vitamin D (as cholecalciferol)	440	I.U.	110
Vitamin E (as d-alpha-tocopherol)	32	I.U.	106
Vitamin K (as phytonadione)	80	mcg	100
Thiamin (as thiamin mononitrate)	4.9	mg	326
Riboflavin	5.6	mg	329
Niacin (as niacinamide)	63	mg	315
Vitamin B_6 (as pyridoxine HCl)	6.5	mg	325
Folate (folic acid)	480	mcg	120
Vitamin B_{12} (as cyanocobalamin)	10	mcg	167
Biotin	360	mcg	120
Pantothenic acid (as D-calcium pantothenate)	12	mg	120
Calcium (as calcium phosphate dibasic)	1,000	mg	100
Iodine (as potassium iodide)	150	mcg	100
Magnesium (as magnesium oxide)	400	mg	100
Zinc (as zinc gluconate)	15	mg	100
Selenium (as selenomethionine)	70	mcg	100
Manganese (as manganese glycinate)	2	mg	100
Chromium (as chromium niacin/glycine chelate)	120	mcg	100
Soy (bean)	2,375	mg	*
90% protein isolate, >2,138mg			
Wheat bran	500	mg	*
Echinacea blend (root, leaf)	100	mg	*
E. purpurea, E. angustifolia			
4% phenolic compounds, 4mg			
Eleuthero (root, Siberian ginseng)	100	mg	*
0.8% eleutherosides, 0.8mg			
Stevia extract (leaf)	10	mg	*
80–85% steviosides, 8–8.5mg			

*Daily value not established.
†Inactive ingredients: oat fiber (as filler).

More About Multi-Boosting Supplements

* **Vitamin A.** This fat-soluble vitamin is necessary for normal vision, healthy mucous membranes (such as those found in the lungs), and a strong, healthy immune response. Vitamin A also provides antioxidant protection for your body.

* **Vitamins B_1, B_2, B_3, B_5, B_6, B_{12}, folic acid,** and **biotin** are all members of the B-complex group and work together to support a healthy nervous system. They also are involved in the transformation of food into usable energy at the cellular level. All B vitamins are water soluble.

* **Vitamin C.** This water-soluble antioxidant vitamin functions in the formation and maintenance of collagen, a protein that *glues* the cells of the body together. It is also necessary in the production of the stress hormones produced by the adrenal glands. Scientific research has proven that vitamin C is a necessary nutritional tool the body uses to maintain a strong immune response and normal healthy healing. As an antioxidant it protects the clear lens and cornea of the eye, and strengthens and protects the walls of blood vessels as well as the interior of every cell in your body.

* **Vitamin D** is necessary for the formation and maintenance of strong healthy bones and teeth. Vitamin D regulates the absorption and use of calcium, a mineral essential to bone structure and strength.

* **Vitamin E.** This powerful antioxidant supports a healthy cardiovascular system and protects brain cells. It also helps stabilize and protect the integrity cell membranes everywhere in the body.

* **Vitamin K** supports normal, healthy blood clotting.

* **Calcium.** This mineral is vital for the formation and maintenance of strong bones. It is one of the nutrients necessary

to support healthy blood pressure levels. In its role as a necessary nutrient for the maintenance of a regular, efficient heartbeat, as well as the movement of nerve impulses, it is called an *electrolyte*.

* **Magnesium.** Like calcium, magnesium is an electrolyte supporting a healthy heartbeat and healthy blood pressure levels. It also supports normal muscle relaxation as well as energy production at the cellular level.

* **Iron.** Without iron, the blood could not move oxygen from the lungs to every cell in your body, and without oxygen, your cells cannot produce energy. Iron also promotes a healthy immune response.

* **Zinc.** This trace mineral is essential for immune function, and the protein synthesis and collagen formation necessary for normal healing and repair. Zinc also supports taste and smell. It is a component of insulin and many vital enzymes, including SOD (superoxide dismutase), a powerful antioxidant produced by your body. Men need extra zinc because they also use it to promote prostate gland function and the production of male sex hormones. So, zinc up, guys!

* **Iodine** is another trace mineral necessary for healthy thyroid function. The thyroid regulates and optimizes the metabolism of food into energy.

* **Selenium** is an antioxidant trace mineral. Selenium works with vitamin E to protect many structures in the body, such as your eyes, lungs, and the walls of your arteries and other blood vessels. In 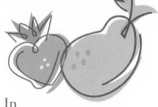 addition, it protects and supports a strong, healthy immune response.

* **Chromium** supports insulin's ability to control blood glucose levels. Chromium also helps activate insulin, which helps

move sugar and fat from the bloodstream into the cell where the sugar and fat can be burned for energy.

* **Soy protein isolate.** In addition to having *isoflavones*, which promote a healthy cardiovascular system and healthy cholesterol levels, soy protein is high in branched-chain amino acids and arginine, which are important to muscle growth. Protein is also vital for the proper healthy repair and reproduction of cells such as those found in bone, skin, hair, and internal organs. Plasma, antibodies, hormones, and enzymes are constructed from amino acids, which are the components of protein. Healthy protein intake also promotes a healthy, strong immune response and mental alertness.

* **Wheat bran** is an insoluble fiber. Wheat bran comes from the outer hull of the seed of wheat grain. Wheat bran optimizes a healthy digestive system, especially the intestines.

* **Echinacea** is a Native American herb that enhances immune cell activity.

* **Eleuthero** (root, Siberian ginseng) is an *adaptogenic* herb. Adaptogens help the body adapt to and protect itself against the side effects of physical, chemical, and biological stress. They also promote physical, mental, and emotional endurance.

Protein Boost™ = Body and Muscle Growth

Our Protein Boost packs a potent punch toward your goal of getting enough powerful protein every day. Added to a smoothie it provides 7 grams of complete vegetarian soy protein, which as part of a diet low in saturated fat and cholesterol may reduce the risk of heart disease. In fact, soy protein has also been linked to

cholesterol reduction, reduced osteoporosis, and overall
hormone balancing. Plus, our Protein Boost includes
all twenty-two amino acids including the nine
essential ones that our bodies cannot manufacture on their own to sustain your body and
build muscle and tissue. In other words, it's a
smoothie kind of good.

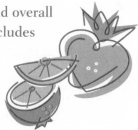

Protein Boost Ingredients Per Serving†
(Serving size: 1 20-cc scoop)

Nutrient	Amount	Unit	%DV
Total protein	7.02	g	14
Soy protein isolate	7,020	mg	*

*Daily value not established.
†Inactive ingredients: none.

More About Protein-Boosting Supplements

✳ **Soy protein isolate** contains plant proteins free of the potentially dangerous saturated fats found in animal sources
of protein. Protein is necessary for building muscle and
is vital for the proper healthy repair and reproduction of
cells such as those found in bone, skin, hair, and internal organs. Plasma, antibodies, hormones, and enzymes are constructed from amino acids, which are the components of
protein. Healthy protein intake also promotes a healthy
strong immune response and mental alertness. Soy protein
has isoflavones, which promote a healthy cardiovascular
system and healthy cholesterol levels. Soy protein is high in
branched-chain amino acids and arginine, which are important to muscle growth.

Vibrant C Boost™ = High-Potency C

Our Vibrant C Boost is steeped in some serious vitamin C folks, in fact 1,000 percent RDI of vitamin C per serving! Why? Studies revealed in *The Real Vitamin & Mineral Book* suggest vitamin C, especially when taken within the range of Optimal Daily Intake of vitamins 1,000 to 5,000 mg, may enhance your immune system and help lessen the symptoms of stress. Extra vitamin C may also help shorten the duration of colds and lessen the severity of cold symptoms. In addition, vitamin C has also been shown to be a powerful antioxidant that protects the body against damage from free radicals (those unstable molecules that try to destroy the integrity or our precious cells). A true vision of overall health, this boost contains Acerola Cherry, a natural form of vitamin C found in cherries; rose hips to protect blood vessels; and citrus *bioflavonoids* that altogether strengthen and protect skin, blood vessels, and internal organs such as lungs and adrenal glands while enabling vitamin C to work more effectively in the body.

Vibrant C Boost Ingredients Per Serving†
(Serving size: ½ teaspoon)

Nutrient	Amount	Unit	%DV
Vitamin C (as ascorbic acid)	600	mg	1,000
Acerola cherry	450	mg	*
Rose hips	300	mg	*
Hesperidin	250	mg	*
Stevia	10	mg	*

*Daily value not established.
†Inactive ingredients: oat fiber (as filler), honey powder (considered a food source), and calcium silicate (as an anticaking agent).

More About Vitamin C–Boosting Supplements

* **Vitamin C** is a powerful antioxidant that protects the interior of cells by neutralizing free radicals. Remember, free radicals are unstable, destructive molecules. Vitamin C also supports the immune system by promoting the healthy production of immune components such a lymphocytes and interferon.
* **Rose hips concentrate.** Rose hips contain generous amounts of bioflavonoids, which work synergistically with vitamin C. Bioflavonoids are particularly helpful in working with vitamin C to protect blood vessels, from the largest arteries and veins to the smallest capillaries.
* **Acerola cherry powder** is generally found within other supplements as a form of vitamin C. Within our formula it boosts the vitamin C level by an additional 25 percent (112.5 mg), while helping to provide a more natural, pleasant taste. Acerola is the tart, cherrylike fruit of a small tree of the West Indies and adjacent areas, used by supplement makers for its high concentrations of vitamin C. FYI: Generally, this fruit is two to four inches in diameter and bright. It is also known as the *Barbados cherry* and *Puerto Rican cherry.*
* **Hesperidin** is a citrus bioflavonoid. Like all bioflavonoids, hesperidin helps vitamin C work more effectively and has antioxidant properties of its own.
* **Honey powder.** Did you know that to produce one pound of honey, bees must bring into the hive seventy-five thousand loads of nectar, or the equivalent of four to six times the circumference of the earth? Honey contains as many as eighty different substances important in human nutrition, including vitamin A, beta-carotene, all

the B-complex vitamins, and vitamins C, D, E, and K. It also contains the minerals magnesium, sulfur, phosphorus, iron, calcium, chlorine, potassium, iodine, sodium, copper, and manganese. Honey also contains a small quantity of an un-known substance that to date science has not been able to synthesize or identify. Here at Jamba, we use honey powder as an additional nutrient as well as a natural sweetener.

✳ **Stevia extract** has a pleasing flavor to help mask some of the vitamin flavors.

Vita Boost™ = Daily Health

For those of you looking for a smoothie kind of way to get your complete set of daily RDIs without taking handfuls of pills, this is your tastiest bet. Why? Our Vita Boost is bursting with 100 percent of your currently recommended vitamin and mineral needs and may also happen to be in total sync with your life! We skip the starches, sugars, and binders found in most supple-ments, and replace them with pure and vital vitamins such as vitamins A, C, D, E, K, and all the Bs for a healthy nervous sys-tem. Plus, Vita Boost contains many vital daily minerals such as magnesium, zinc, calcium, and selenium to protect your eyes, lungs, arteries, and blood vessels.

Vita Boost Ingredients Per Serving[†]
(Serving size: 1 teaspoon)

Nutrient	Amount	Unit	%DV
Vitamin A (as retinyl palmitate)	5,000	I.U.	100
Vitamin C (as ascorbic acid)	66	mg	110
Vitamin D (as cholecalciferl)	440	I.U.	110
Vitamin E (as d-alpha-tocopherol)	32	I.U.	106
Vitamin K (as phytonadione)	80	mcg	100

Nutrient	Amount	Unit	%DV
Thiamin (as thiamin mononitrate)	4.9	mg	326
Riboflavin	5.6	mg	329
Niacin (as niacinamide)	63	mg	315
Vitamin B$_6$ (as pyridoxine HCl)	6.5	mg	325
Folate (folic acid)	480	mcg	120
Vitamin B$_{12}$ (as cyanocobalamin)	10	mcg	167
Biotin	360	mcg	120
Pantothenic acid (as D-calcium pantothenate)	12	mg	120
Calcium (as calcium carbonate)	1,000	mg	100
Iodine (as potassium iodide)	150	mcg	100
Magnesium (as magnesium oxide)	400	mg	100
Zinc (as zinc gluconate)	15	mg	100
Selenium (as selenomethionine)	70	mcg	100
Manganese (as manganese glycinate)	2	mg	100
Chromium (as chromium niacin/ glycine chelate)	120	mcg	100
Stevia extract (leaf)	10	mg	*
80–85% steviosides, 8–8.5mg			

*Daily value not established.
†Inactive ingredients: none.

More About Vitamin-Boosting Supplements

* **Vitamin A** is a fat-soluble vitamin necessary for normal vision, healthy mucous membranes, such as those found in the lungs, and a strong, healthy immune response. Vitamin A also provides antioxidant protection for your body.
* **Vitamins B$_1$, B$_2$, B$_3$, B$_5$, B$_6$, B$_{12}$, folic acid,** and **biotin** are all members of the B-complex group and work together to support a healthy nervous system. They also help turn food into usable energy at the cellular level.
* **Vitamin C** functions in the formation and maintenance of

collagen, a protein that *glues* the cells of the body together, as well as the stress hormones produced by the adrenal glands. Scientific research has proven that vitamin C is a necessary nutritional tool the body uses to maintain a strong immune response and normal healthy healing. As an antioxidant vitamin C helps protect the clear lens and cornea of the eye, and strengthens and protects the walls of blood vessels as well as the interior of every cell in your body.

* **Vitamin D** is necessary for the formation and maintenance of strong, healthy bones and teeth. Vitamin D regulates the absorption and use of calcium, a mineral essential to bone structure and strength.

* **Vitamin E** is a powerful antioxidant that supports a healthy cardiovascular system and protects brain cells. It also helps stabilize and protect the integrity cell membranes everywhere in the body.

* **Vitamin K** supports normal, healthy blood clotting.

* **Calcium** is a mineral vital for the formation and maintenance of strong bones.

* **Magnesium** is an electrolyte supporting a healthy heartbeat and healthy blood pressure levels. It also supports normal muscle relaxation as well as energy production at the cellular level.

* **Zinc** is a trace mineral essential for immune function, and the protein synthesis and collagen formation necessary for normal healing and repair. Zinc also supports taste and smell. It is associated with insulin and many vital enzymes and protective antioxidants. Men need extra zinc because it promotes prostate gland function and the production of male sex hormones.

* **Iodine** is necessary for healthy thyroid function. The thyroid regulates and optimizes the metabolism of food into energy.

✳ **Selenium** works with vitamin E to protect many structures in the body, such as your eyes, lungs, and the walls of your arteries and other blood vessels. In addition, it protects and supports a strong, healthy immune response.

✳ **Chromium.** This is a *chelated* (bonded) form of the trace mineral chromium that is extremely bioavailable. Chromium supports insulin's ability to control blood glucose levels. Chromium also helps activates insulin, which helps move sugar and fat from the bloodstream in order to be burned for energy.

Burner Boost™ = Diet Complement

Our Burner Boost is featured as part of our Kiwi Berry Burner functional smoothie to complement the low fat content and great nutrition of all Jamba Juice's smoothies. This metabolism-boosting formula may help inhibit the body's ability to store fat, while the special botanicals and insoluble fiber may help control appetite. Burner Boost has been scientifically designed to help in your weight maintenance program and along with sensible eating and becoming more active, it may help keep you fit and trim!

Burner Boost Ingredients Per Serving†
(Serving size: ½ teaspoon)

Nutrient	Amount	Unit	%DV
Garcinia cambogia (fruit)	500	mg	*
50% hydroxycitric acid, 250mg			

Nutrient	Amount	Unit	%DV
Guggul (gum)	138	mg	*
2.5% guggulsterone, 3.5mg			
Triphala (blend of the following):	84	mg	*
Terminalia chebula (fruit)			
Terminalia belerica (fruit)			
Emblica officinalis (fruit)			
Chromium (as chromium picolinate)	120	mcg	100
Guarana (seed)			
10% caffeine, 20mg	200	mg	*
Stevia extract (leaf)			
80–85% steviosides, 8–8.5mg	10	mg	*

*Daily value not established.
†Inactive ingredients: oat fiber (as filler).

More About Metabolism-Boosting Supplements

✳ **Citrin** is the registered trademark name for the botanical extract from the fruit of the *Garcinia cambogia* tree from India. *Garcinia cambogia* is grown in southern India, and its active ingredient is something called *hydroxycitric acid* (HCA). *Garcinia cambogia* fruit has a long history as a flavoring agent and food preservative. (The Sabinsa Corporation sells a derivative of *Garcinia cambogia* under the trademarked name Citrin® and has also created a patented version called Citrin® K.) HCA helps the liver control the conversion of sugar into fat. HCA may also help control appetite. If used in conjunction with a weight program that includes a healthy diet and reasonably restricted caloric intake, as well as exercise, HCA can help the body manage sugar in a healthy way, maintain a normal health control of appetite, and decrease the body's production of fat.

✳ **Guggul** (or 2.5 percent *gugglesterones*) is the gum resin extracted from the bark of a small spiny tree that grows in arid, rocky parts of India and Arabia. This Ayurvedic (a holistic system of medicine that originated in India five thousand years ago) herb helps support thyroid gland activity.

✳ **Triphala** is another product based on the ancient art of Ayurvedic medicine. It is a modern blending of three different fruit-based ingredients—*Terminalia chebula, Terminalia belerica,* and *Emblica officinalis.* Triphala can be found in capsules and powder form and has been shown to help support a healthy metabolism and help promote normal cholesterol levels.

✳ **Chromium** (picolinate) can be found in capsule form. It is a chelated (bonded) form of the trace mineral chromium, which is extremely bioavailable. Chromium supports insulin's ability to control blood glucose levels. Chromium also helps activate insulin, which helps move sugar and fat from the bloodstream into the cell, where the sugar and fat can be burned for energy.

✳ **Guarana** is a South American herb that is a natural source of caffeine, which acts as a central nervous system stimulant and increases metabolism. It can be found in tablet and powder form.

✳ **Citrus aurantium** is known more commonly as bitter orange. Bitter orange is often used to help relieve nausea and soothe the stomach from troubles such as gas, indigestion, and bloating. Studies indicate that extracts of Citrus aurantium may increase your metabolic rate, or *thermogenesis*—the production of body heat in the muscles and fat—without affecting heart rate or blood pressure and stimulate the breakdown of fat. Simultaneously, this stimulation causes an increase in your metabolic rate, which may help you burn more calories. Citrus aurantium may also act as an appetite suppressant. Currently, you can find this extract within other supplements.

✳ **Gingerroot powder** helps soothe the stomach, control appetite, and relieve gas. In its most natural state, gingerroot can be found in many supermarkets nationwide. At home ginger can be used to enhance the flavors of many dishes. As a food additive, ginger can be found in things such as candy, pastries, tea, and, yes, ginger ale. In botanical terms, ginger is known as *Zingiber officinale*. It has been grown and used for thousands of years in China and India. Many consider ginger a food, as it contains protein, carbohydrates, fat, calcium, phosphorus, iron, sodium, and potassium. As a supplement, ginger can be found as a root powder, and in capsule form.

✳ **Stevia extract** has a sweet flavor that helps mask some harsh botanical flavors.

Now you have a basic understanding of how power foods, along with power fruits and Jamba Boosts, may help you achieve your nutritional goals. Later, and step-by-step in my 21-Day Smoothie and Juice Guide I will explain even more benefits to choosing power foods over empty calorie foods, and show you many ways to adopt them into your daily life without any aggravation whatsoever.

Chapter 3

Preparing for 21 Days of Success

Shopping for Power Fruits, Vegetables, Foods, and Supplements

Okay, the moment has almost arrived for you to begin the adventure of your lifetime. But before I take you down the aisles of your local grocery and health-food stores to buy the most powerful fruits, vegetables, other foods, supplements, and equipment you'll need, take a look at what you already have at home. Begin with the refrigerator. Open it and look inside. Is there anything that's been sitting for way too long? Are there any junk foods that need to be tossed out? If so, trash the stale items you know aren't good for you.

Now go to your cupboards. Take a good look. How many products can you find that have too many saturated fats or empty calories? If you feel comfortable, throw them out now. If the items have not been opened, consider taking them to a shelter. Look carefully at the cooking oils you currently have. Have any reached their expiration dates? Do any smell funky? If so, toss 'em. The best oils to keep on hand are olive oil and canola, which we will discuss in greater detail during week two of my guide.

In case you're not sure whether you should toss something, let's talk about one of the most important things you need to do to become healthier and stay that way: *Read food labels.* On the back or side of virtually every package of food or beverage there is a food label that lists all the ingredients, as well as the nutritional values. Try to get used to reading all food labels *before* you buy anything in the future. Knowing what something is made of, how many overall calories it has, and how many grams of saturated fats are in it can help you take control of your weight and your health—for good. At first reading labels may seem a little complicated, but in the long run, it will be worth your while.

Grab a package of food right now and let's go over it together. Look on the package until you find a label that reads "Nutrition Facts." At the top of the nutrition facts label it tells you what *one* serving size is. It is very important to understand what one serving size is. Generally, one serving size is a heck of a lot smaller than what we actually eat. For instance, if one serving size of candy has 200 calories . . . and we eat three times that amount . . . we just ate 600 calories!

1 serving = 200 calories x 3 (amount we really ate) = 600 calories

Follow the food label down or around until you find a section that lists the nutrients. By now, you know a balance of key nutrients is important for overall health. Look at the label again. Notice the first group is stuff that you should limit or avoid eating too much of, such as saturated fat, cholesterol, and sodium. Why? Because eating too much fat or sodium may increase your risk of many chronic diseases such as heart disease, certain cancers, and high blood pressure. Eating too many calories can lead to becoming overweight or obese. This section also includes important nutrients such as potassium, carbohydrates, fiber, sugars, calcium, iron, protein, and vitamins. Getting the right amount of these nutrients in your diet can greatly improve your health and help reduce your risk of getting many diseases.

On the nutrition facts label, the nutrients are usually broken down for us into something called Percent Daily Value (%DV), which simply means the percentage of daily nutrients governmental experts believe we should be getting from the foods we eat on a daily basis. As for power foods—namely, carbs, proteins, and fats—the recommended daily percentages based on an average 2,000 calorie a day diet, work out to be:

Calories	2,000 = 100%
Carbs	55–60%
Protein	10–20%
Fats	20–30%

Of course, if you hate math, don't worry. The label does most of the math for you. In fact, it actually breaks the nutrients down into a series of percentages based on the average need to get 2,000 calories a day, set by government labeling guidelines.

By looking at the %DV of a nutrient you can quickly tell if the amount is high or low. It may contain 10 percent fiber or 30 percent saturated fat. Each day you want to achieve 100 percent of all the important nutrients such as calcium, iron, and vitamins A and C, while trying to limit your intake of certain things like saturated fat and cholesterol to less than 100 percent DV.

Let's continue down the label . . .

Sugar and protein: Notice that sugar and protein are not broken down into a percentage of daily value. As we mentioned in Chapter 2, the FDA has not firmly established a value for sugar

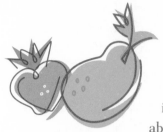 or protein yet. Although some health experts, including the USDA, recommend you limit your refined sugar intake to about 40 grams (not including milk or fruit sugar), or less than 15 percent of your overall caloric intake. You may also need to get an average of about 50 grams of low-fat protein each day.

Salt or sodium: Most experts, including the USDA, recommend you keep your sodium intake to less than 2,400 milligrams.

Calcium: Sometimes the calcium section is broken down into %DVs and sometimes it isn't. Most experts suggest teens consume about 1,300 mg and postmenopausal women 1,200 mg. For most other adults it's 1,000 mg. As always, when in doubt ask your doctor.

Near the bottom of the nutrition facts label you will find a list of the actual ingredients that it took to create the actual product. Find two other products in your cupboard and look at the ingredients. Isn't it amazing how many strange chemicals and colorings are listed?

From today forward try to buy more products with natural and basic ingredients on the label that you recognize, rather than a long list of complicated chemicals and artificial colors. Be especially aware of products containing hydrogenated and partially hydrogenated oils, which form something called trans-fatty acids. Science tells us that saturated fats and trans-fatty acids raise bad cholesterol (LDL) and put us at greater risk for heart attacks and other diseases. That's why health professionals tell us to limit our saturated-fat intake to less than 20 grams a day, about 10 percent of our total daily calories, or about a third of your overall fat intake. We will fully explore this topic later in my guide.

Okay, now that your refrigerator and cupboards are a little barer . . . let's go buy some healthy things to fill them back up again!

General Tips for Buying Power Foods at the Grocery Store

Dairy Power

✳ Stick with nonfat, low-fat, or 1 percent fat products. If you are used to eating or drinking "whole" dairy products, ease into it as slowly as you'd like. Keep reminding yourself that after you succeed at twenty-one days of switching to something more nutritious, you will become totally accustomed to it. In fact, you will get so used to the taste that you will actually think a dairy product tastes strange if it has too much "whole" milk in it.

✳ Go for cheeses with less fat, such as low-fat mozzarella, part-skim Ricotta, and Swiss. Again, the saturated-fat content is right there on the label.

✳ Buy as much yogurt as you and your family can possibly eat in a week. Go for the low-fat versions, and choose "plain" varieties or yogurts with less sugar if you can handle the taste.

✳ As far as eggs go, if you can find them, try some eggs fortified with omega-3 fats, the good kind of essential fatty acids found in fish, such as salmon. Buy "organic" eggs, if you like. Organic eggs are generally produced without the use of growth hormones, antibiotics, or toxic pesticides. Or go for the "free range" eggs. At least those hens get to run around outdoors! Just remember to watch out for cholesterol. One egg weighing in at 215 mg of cholesterol has almost a full day's RDI of cholesterol in it (300 mg a day is optimal). So make more omelets with egg whites!

✳ Buy some low-fat cottage cheese to enjoy for lunch, snack time, or as a side dish at suppertime.

✳ Try a small container of rice milk or anything made with soy! Many health experts believe soy products may be preferable to cow's milk because your body is better equipped to absorb more calcium from a plant-based soy product.

Power Proteins and Meats

* Choose to buy lean meat. If the meat you buy does have fat, trim it off before eating. Not only does this reduce your fat intake, but the FDA tells us that the residue of certain pesticides concentrates in the animal fat.
* Try one meat-free product. Garden burgers and meatless corn dogs are in the frozen section. Most of them taste great.
* Buy some fresh or frozen fish, preferably wild Pacific salmon, farm-raised trout, croaker, farm-raised catfish, and tilapia, all of which generally contain the lowest levels of mercury, according to the Environmental Working Group, a Washington-based consumer organization.
* More words of cautionary fish tales? Try not to eat more than one serving per month of canned tuna, blue mussel, Eastern oyster, cod, pollock, mahimahi, Great Lakes salmon, Gulf Coast blue crab, channel catfish, and lake whitefish because of possible high levels of mercury.
* Other *good* choices include Atlantic blue crab, flounder (summer), haddock, or shrimp. Again, the omega-3 fatty acids in fish can help reduce the risk of heart disease, so if you don't eat fish regularly, as in a couple of times a week, you may wish to take a supplement featuring omega-3 fatty acids.
* Read the labels of processed fish products carefully. Sometimes those tasty little fish sticks are nothing more than frozen fatty chemical pops.
* Also, pregnant women should completely avoid tuna steaks, sea bass, Gulf Coast oysters, halibut, marlin, walleye, pike, white croaker, and largemouth bass, says the EWG. And, current U.S. recommendations urge you to limit your fish

consumption to no more than 12 ounces per week due to mercury content.

Power Fruits

* When shopping for fruits, look for the richest in color. It's best to select fruits that are on the verge of ripeness rather than those that appear too immature. The riper the fruit, the more nutrients it has inside. Watch out for bruises, though. Buy a wide variety of colors, sizes, and shapes. Think: bananas, strawberries, blueberries, apples, oranges, and any other fruits in season that look delicious to you.
* Try to buy organic because these products are grown without pesticides and in a way that is designed to help protect the environment, pollute less, and promote good health. Plus, they often taste better.
* Freezing fruit is one of the best methods for enjoying fruit all year long. You can buy assorted packs of berries that thaw out in minutes and can be added to yogurt and cereals year round!
* Canned fruits can be good too. Check labels and choose fruits packed in less sugar and sodium.

FACT FUNFASTFACT FUNFASTFACT FUNFASTFACT FUNFASTFACT
UNFASTFACT FUNFASTFACT FUNFASTFACT FUNFASTFACT FUNFA

Want the men in your life to stay healthy? Bring on the smoothies, sister! Middle-aged and senior men who eat little fruit are 46 percent more likely to develop high blood pressure over the next four years than guys who eat five servings of fruit a day, according to a recent Harvard study.

Power Vegetables

* Just as in choosing fruits, select vegetables that appear rich in color. Opt for a wide, colorful variety.
* Choose as many prewashed, precut veggies as you like. When something is easy to prepare or can be snacked on straight out of the bag you will be much more likely to choose a healthy low-fat, high-fiber vegetable over a bag of overprocessed treats.
* Buy more broccoli, asparagus, and dark green leafy vegetables.
* Choose more purple cabbages and eggplant.
* Grab a couple of artichokes and some sugar snap peas!
* Try a new vegetable every week if you like.
* Don't be afraid of frozen vegetables. Often they are flash-frozen immediately after being picked so they retain many important nutrients.
* Stock up on a few vegetable soups that sound tantalizing to you. Check the labels. Buy soups with less salt and fewer strange, artificial ingredients.

Power Nuts

* Buy an assortment of raw nuts such as whole almonds, walnuts, Brazil nuts, cashews, and hazelnuts. Nuts are a great source of healthy oils (omega-3 and monounsaturated). Plus, most are full of fiber, protein, potassium, magnesium, selenium, and vitamin E. If you've only had them roasted and salted in the past, you may be surprised at how different, and yet utterly *delicious*, raw nuts can taste.
* Buy natural peanut butter. It tastes delicious, and a spoonful of it along with a ripe apple can be all you need to eat an hour before a workout.

Power Oils

✳ Go for extra-virgin olive oil. Olive oil tastes fantastic and is rich in monounsaturated fats, which may help raise good cholesterol slightly. Dab your bread in olive oil instead of butter, and your heart will practically leap out and applaud!

✳ Reach for a bottle of canola oil. Did you know canola oil was created by Canadian agronomists (agricultural scientists) using a special strain of the rapeseed plant bred to be superior nutritionally? Hence, the word *canola* is a blend of the words *Canadian* and *oil*. In fact, more than 60 percent of canola oil is rich in heart-healthy monounsaturated fats.

✳ Look for products that contain flaxseeds in any form, including oils and seeds. Flaxseeds are bursting with those amazing omega-3 oils that help control heart disease risk and diabetes. Plus, they are teeming with fiber, iron, protein, and even potassium. You can also add flaxseed oil to any smoothie or sprinkle a few ground seeds on your yogurt or whole-wheat cereal in the morning.

Power Breads, Grains, and Cereals

✳ Read all labels. Only buy breads that list the word *whole* as the *first* ingredients, such as *whole* wheat, *whole* bran, and *whole* oats. You will be very surprised to learn that many types of bread that claim *healthy* or even *whole* on the package are not as healthy as they could be. Remember, every time a manufacturer refines a whole-wheat product, the most important nutrients are lost only to be replaced by a few *fortified* ingredients to make them seem healthier than they actually are!

* Also, look for cereals that contain *whole* as the first ingredient.
* If a product uses the term *good source* of a certain nutrient, it simply means that one serving contains between 10 to 19 percent of the RDI for that particular nutrient.
* Buy more brown and wild rice. The more natural the better; however, instant brown rice is infinitely better for your body than white rice. Remember, white rice and other refined grains have been stripped of almost all of their nutrients.

Power Drinks

* If possible skip buying sodas. Instead, pick up a bottled brand of herbal, green, or regular iced tea with as little sugar as you can handle. Because many bottled iced teas may contain as much added refined sugars as a soda, buy boxed teas and make your own enticing brew. Herbal teas come in many delicious flavors and you can enjoy them with or without adding any sugar. Black and green teas, which have about half the caffeine coffee does, also come in all sorts of tasty new varieties. I really like the spiced versions.
* Buy 100 percent juice whenever possible. If OJ is your favorite, buy it with the pulp. Without the pulp juice has less fiber. The more fiber, the more it is considered a complex carb, which, if you remember, gives you more energy.
* Go for juices that are also made with *less sugar* or *no sugars added.* Most of them taste great!
* Enjoy more 100 percent berry juices. One glass of strawberry, cherry, blueberry—or any other berry, for that matter—juice has been shown in studies to reduce a woman's risk of urinary tract infection by more than a third, because berries contain flavonols, which help prevent bacteria from sticking to your cells. Plus, berries contain lots of antioxidants shown to reduce the risk of many cancers.
* Look for a 100 percent vegetable juice that you can enjoy,

such as tomato or fresh carrot. Read the labels and find one with the least amount of sodium and artificial ingredients.

* If you buy bottled juices in a grocery store, I recommend juices that have been pasteurized similar to the juice concentrates that we use in some of our smoothies. In Jamba Juice stores, the fresh squeezed juices are unpasteurized, but we have created our own standards to ensure the safety and integrity of our products.

* If drinking alcohol is not a problem for you and not against your religion, buy a nice bottle of heart-healthy red wine, perhaps a lovely Merlot, Shiraz, or a full-bodied Cabernet Sauvignon (and a wine opener, if you don't have one). Studies have revealed that many of the same antioxidants found in grape juice are even more abundant in red wine.

* If you enjoy the hearty taste of malt and barley in beer, choose a *light* variety, and try not to overindulge.

* Many researchers now believe that moderate drinking of red wine may help keep the blood flowing through your veins more easily. Always remember, however, that moderate drinking is the key.

* How do experts define *moderate drinking*? Moderate is defined as a maximum of one drink per day for women and two for men. One drink is technically classified as 12 ounces of beer, 5 ounces of wine, or 1.5 ounces (a shot) of hard liquor, such as vodka, gin, and tequila. Do not save up your daily quota for the weekend! And remember, drinking too much may kill brain cells, damage your liver, and increase your risk of many cancers, such as breast, mouth, and liver.

* Confused about all the new "designer waters" flooding the market? Liquids with names like "Glaceau Vitaminwater," "MaxO$_2$," or even divine-sounding ones such as "Acqua della Madonna," a water imported from a two-thousand-year-old spring south of Naples, Italy, often referred to as "The choice of popes, emperors, and other dignitaries for

centuries!" Well, it's no wonder you may be mystified, there are hundreds of wild waters to choose from! So what's the skinny? Designer waters are simply cool-sounding drinks, often fortified with vitamins, minerals, botanicals, as well as other strange flavors, colors, and added sugars. How do you pick a nutritional winner? *Read the labels.* Try ones with fewer *empty calories* than, say, a soda. As you will discover, some waters are much healthier than others as far as added sugars, caffeine, and salt are concerned.

Powerfully Good Seasonings

∗ Buy plenty of garlic, ginger, onions, and cayenne pepper to flavor your foods.
∗ Experiment with fresh herbs such as dill and basil, which can be chopped and added to salads, dressings, and many meat dishes.

Power Soups

∗ Homemade soups are the best; however, for those pressed for time there are many healthy canned choices as well. Try a vegetarian lentil, black bean, split pea, vegetable, or even chicken barley. Again, check the labels for saturated fats, added sugars, and sodium levels.

Tips for Buying Power Supplements

Although most of us try to eat healthfully all the time, few of us actually do. It can be tough sometimes, I know. That's why taking supplements, especially a multivitamin complete with minerals every day is a great starting point. At a cost of about ten cents a day you can ensure that your precious body will get more of the nutrients it needs to stay healthy. In fact, according to many experts, including the American Cancer Society, the FDA, and the Council for Responsible Nutrition, taking multivitamins and other key supplements on a regular basis can promote good health and help prevent disease. Research has shown that using multivitamins, especially those with minerals, and other single-nutrient supplements, such as calcium and folic acid, can do amazing things—ranging from boosting your immune system to drastically reducing the risk of certain birth defects. However, the American Heart Association reminds us that all nutrients may be potentially toxic if ingested in massive quantities over long periods of time. So don't overdo it in the supplement department.

Additional supplements should be carefully chosen based on your stage in life, your gender, and the kind of lifestyle you lead. For example, calcium is important for all men and women, but it is especially critical for growing children who are still building bone mass and seniors seeking to preserve it. Athletes need more calories, especially complex carbs, than the rest of us. In case you are worried about safety, relax. Most dietary supplements are regulated by the protective agency of the Food and Drug Administration, which recently passed a law that will make supplements even safer in the years to come.

Don't forget, the world of supplements is an ongoing science. Supplements should be taken *in addition* to a healthful diet. Supplements do not have the power to take a lousy diet and miraculously transform it into an Olympic athlete's diet! In fact, the American Heart Association urges us that vitamin and mineral supplements should *not* be used as a substitute for a more balanced, nutritious diet, one that is low in saturated fat, trans-fat, cholesterol, and limits excess calories.

Along with eating well-balanced foods and becoming as active as possible, supplements are for those who yearn to blossom into even healthier, happier, sexier human beings. Why? Vitamins, minerals, herbs, and botanicals can help counteract the stresses in our lives. They can help make up for lost nutrients from foods grown from depleted soils. They can help us look better and feel younger. They can give us more energy and help us handle stress more efficiently. Like most things that involve your health, it's best to ask your doctor for advice on exactly which supplements are best for you. Or you may want to seek out a highly trained clinical nutritionist to help design a supplement program that is right for *you*. How do you find someone qualified? Your best bet on individualized nutrition counseling is to find a registered dietician (R.D.), all of whom have been certified by the Commission on Dietetic Registration. To find an R.D. near you, call the American Dietetic Association at 800-366-1655, or get a referral in your area from a doctor or a friend.

Remember, there is no legal definition for the term *nutritionist*. So anyone can theoretically call himself or herself a nutritionist with little to no specialized training, or even a license. There are legal definitions for the terms *dietitian, registered dietitian,* and *dietitian/nutritionist*, however, so for your safety seek out an R.D. or an M.D.!

What to Look For in a Basic Multivitamin
A good multivitamin should provide 100 percent of the generally accepted governmental Daily Value for all or at least *most* of the thirteen key vitamins (glance back at the RDI chart on pages 18–19). Read labels. The %DV can be found in the supplement facts box. You may also want to buy vitamins promising potency such as those listing *high performance, extra potent, complete, megavitamins,* and *rich in antioxidants.* You may also want to try those *one-a-day multinutrient* packages that have four or more supplements inside.

What to Look For in a Multivitamin with Minerals

A multivitamin with minerals should provide you with 100 percent of your daily value for all or most vitamins and many important minerals. FYI: Most will not give you enough calcium. You probably need at least 1,000 mg of calcium in your diet, and little pills are just that—too small to contain 100 percent of your vitamin and mineral needs plus calcium. So you may want to take additional calcium supplements.

When to Take Supplements

Vitamins and minerals work best when you take them along with a meal or a nutritious smoothie and a light snack. Why? This combination increases your body's chances of absorbing more of the nutrients. It also means you will have less gas, less heartburn, and less indigestion than if you popped a supplement on an empty stomach. Take supplements a few minutes before a light meal, during it, or up to a half hour afterward. Remember, you can only absorb so many nutrients at a time. To increase your body's ability to maximize the power of more than one supplement, take them at different mealtimes during the day.

The Most Important Individual Supplements

* **Vitamin E** protects the heart by preventing the waxy buildup of plaque in your arteries caused by bad cholesterol (LDL) oxidizing, and may protect against prostate and colon cancer. Vitamin E has also been shown to protect your brain from the debilitating effects of Alzheimer's disease. Vitamins C and E, when taken together regularly along with a multivitamin, have been shown to decrease the development of cataracts by up to 60 percent. And although vitamin E can

help prevent heart disease, it can also decrease the benefits of some cholesterol-lowering drugs (statins). So if you are on a cholesterol-lowering drug, please consult a doctor.

* **Vitamin C** protects your immune system and may reduce the risk of many stomach and bladder cancers. Researchers also found that when vitamin C is taken with vitamin E supplements the brain functions better for longer periods of time and the chance of getting dementia in old age is reduced greatly.

* **Calcium.** You probably know that calcium is good for your bones, teeth, and gums. But did you know that calcium may also: help your heart beat regularly; lower bad (LDL) cholesterol; help muscles grow; prevent cancer; lower blood pressure; provide energy; and help break down fats so your body can use them as energy? Also, for the lactose intolerant, you may not be getting enough calcium in your diet, which can lead to osteoporosis (bone degeneration), so you may want to take calcium supplements.

* **B vitamins** including folic acid—help protect against birth defects. Because most pregnancies are a surprise, the Nutrition Board of the Institute of Medicine recommends that all women who may get pregnant get 0.4 mg of folic acid daily. Also, pregnant women who do not consume enough folic acid—a vitamin that is found in many fruits and vegetables and is often added to enriched flour—are at a higher risk of giving birth to babies with problems such as neural tube defects. And because folic acid is needed at the very beginning of pregnancy, some experts suggest folic acid supplements even for those women who could become pregnant, just to make sure they are safe.

* **Lutein** is one of the most important antioxidants your eye has to combat free radicals. Getting enough lutein has been shown to help prevent seniors from going blind, especially

from a disease called *age-related macular degeneration*. Lutein has recently been added to many high-performance multivitamins, and you can also find it in capsule form.

* **Omega-3 fatty acids** (such as EPA and DHA) have been shown to prolong life by protecting against heart disease. Nowadays, you can find it in single supplement capsules or added to a multivitamin. Omega-3 fatty acid can also be found naturally in flaxseeds and walnuts.

* **Vitamin D.** If you spend too little of your time outdoors, you may need extra vitamin D that your skin makes naturally when it is exposed to sunlight. Generally, ten to fifteen minutes of daily sunlight without SPF protection is enough.

* **Vitamin B$_{12}$.** Some seniors may be deficient in vitamin B$_{12}$, because aging can cause many of them to lose their ability to absorb B$_{12}$ from the foods they eat.

In addition, the FDA tells us those rare vitamin deficiency diseases such as scurvy, pellagra, and beriberi do occur very infrequently. Those who may need a little more than the minimum amount of vitamins and minerals, for example, to correct a deficiency disease as diagnosed by your doctor, may require doses that are ten to sometimes a thousand times stronger than the RDI of a nutrient. That's when special supplements and our line of Jamba Boosts may be even more helpful.

One more *dose* of *mega* caution: The following short list of supplements may be harmful if taken in excessive doses: vitamin A, niacin, vitamin B$_6$, vitamin D, iron, and folic acid, according to the Food and Nutrition Science Alliance. Other very recent studies done by the Nutrition Center at Tufts University have shown that excessive amounts of vitamin E supplementation may increase the risk of heart attacks and strokes and that iron overload may increase the risk of heart disease. So always consult your doctor before beginning any diet, supplement, or exercise program. Lastly, keep all vitamins, minerals, and supplements in a nice and cool, dry and dark space such as a kitchen cupboard—out of a child's reach! Supplements should not see the light of day. Sunlight drains them of their antioxidizing powers.

Equipment Needs

Before you begin your twenty-one-day journey, there are some important pieces of equipment you will need to purchase.

✳ **Blender.** First on your list of "things to buy" is a blender. If you already have one, chances are it isn't powerful enough to blend smoothies with the right texture and viscosity of the Jamba Juice at-home versions that you and your family will be enjoying for years to come. When selecting a blender, look for the highest-quality, most powerful blender you can afford. Your new blending tool should have at least two to three horsepower. Sure a forty-dollar, one-half horsepower model can blend a few beverages fairly well *for a while*; however, to get the same thick texture and silky viscosity of a Jamba Juice smoothie you will need to get a blender that features precision engineering and advanced blade design and is strong enough to last for your newer, longer, healthier haul!

Two brands of blenders I recommend are Vita-Mix® and Blendtec®. Vita-Mix is an innovative leader in the marketplace and carries some of the highest-quality commercial and at-home blenders in the world. Blendtec is another high-quality line of blenders. Many of their models are fast, easy, and powerful. You can even chop small portions of nuts or make savory soups, sauces, and salad dressings with many of their models. For more info, check out the On-line Blenders and Juicers (see page 229).

*   **Juicer.** For overall juicing I also recommend buying the very best. Much like a spouse, you want to find a juicer with style, strength, and endurance. There are many good-quality models out there to choose from; however, the two brands I recommend are Omega® and Acme®. Most Omega juicers are powerful, priced reasonably, and easy to use. The Omega 4000, for instance, is a great choice because it's easier to use and clean than most other juice extractors on the market. In addition, because pulp is extracted into a totally separate container, you can juice gallons of energizing liquids without emptying the pulp collector every five minutes.

One of the models I like is the Acme Juicerator because it's strong, reliable, and converts fresh fruits and vegetables into rich, pure juice almost instantly. What better way is there to obtain the essential nutrients from fresh foods? Plus, unlike some cheaper blenders that grind food into a messy clump, the Juicerator cleanly separates the juice from the pulp. And because the Acme Juicerator can extract almost every last drop of moisture from fruits and vegetables, it produces a juice far richer and tastier than you may have ever experienced so far.

For more information, see On-line Blenders and Juices, page 229.

Exercise Needs

Becoming more active is one of the most important things you can do to ensure better health, stave off future diseases, *and* boost your sex appeal. When you work out, brain chemicals, such as endorphins, adrenaline, serotonin, and dopamine, are increased, which in turn can boost your mood! In fact, when those natural "feel good" chemicals are boosted through exer-

cise your self-esteem may heighten. You may feel more pleasure. You may feel more alert. Exercise also helps combat the
effects of stress and may help you sleep better.

Becoming more fit may also improve your love life. Oxy-
genated blood may flow more effectively to vital sexual organs.
The extra levels of serotonin released may improve your "mood"
to get busy between the sheets. Plus, when your body becomes
more toned, your buns and thighs firmer, you will probably feel
a whole lot sexier. Think about it: Would you rather sleep with
an athlete or a couch potato? Thought so.

So if you really want to become healthier, happier, and sexier . . . *regular exercise is a must.* I am not asking you to follow
some horrible exercise program you hate. I am suggesting you
find activities that *you* like, schedule a time of the day that fits
into *your* schedule, and get busy. When exercise is fun and
convenient for you, you will be more apt to continue working
out long into the future. I will get more into this subject during my 21-Day Plan. Until then, here's what you need to get
started:

* **Shoes.** Before you begin the 21-Day Plan, go to a sporting
  goods store and buy yourself at least one pair of running,
  walking, or multipurpose shoes. Look for sales, but don't
  buy a pair of exercise shoes just because they are cheap. You
  need at least one pair of sneakers that feel extremely good
  and very comfortable *for you.* Buy a few pairs of good-quality
  athletic socks too.
* **Activewear.** While you're at the sporting goods store, check
  out their selection of comfortable jogging pants, shorts, sports
  bras, jock straps, and even entire sporty ensembles. No matter
  what size you are now, you will feel a lot better wearing something that fits well and has a zing of contemporary flair to it.
* **Weights.** Next, look at the dumbbells. Strength training is
  an important part of overall fitness, which I will fully ex-

plain during my 21-Day Guide, so ask a salesperson to help you find an affordable pair of very light dumbbells (stick with the one- to five-pound models) to begin.

* **Your choice.** Browse on your own for a while. Look at all the various pieces of sporting equipment. When you were a kid did you enjoy softball, swimming, bicycling, basketball, jump rope, volleyball, or playing Frisbee? Buy a softball and a pair of baseball gloves for you and a friend to play catch during breaks at work. Or buy a new swimsuit and a pair of goggles so you can go for early-morning swims when the mood strikes you. Or pick up a couple of Frisbees to throw around during your lunch hour. In other words, look for sporting equipment that looks fun to you and buy it!

* **Compare.** If you are a homebody, you may also want to look at their selection of high-end treadmills, stationary bikes, and stair climbers. Stationary equipment is fantastic for working out at home . . . if you use the machine! Generally, these items are very expensive. Don't buy it if you will not use it. Jot down a few prices. When you get home, go on line and see if you can get a better deal.

Body/Mind/Spirit Needs— Music, Candles, and Books

* **Music.** Along with eating a colorful variety of healthier foods and becoming more active, music can also help motivate you to achieve your goals. One song on the radio, for instance, can turn a dreary morning into a delightful day. A fast-paced or inspirational piece of music playing on your headphones can make you yearn to fly like an eagle.

FACT FUNFASTFACT FUNFASTFACT FUNFASTFACT FUNFASTFACT
UNFASTFACT FUNFASTFACT FUNFASTFACT FUNFASTFACT FUNFA

Listening to music has been shown to have many benefits
including increasing your chances of scoring better on a
test just by listening to ten minutes of music right before
you take it! More music to your ears? Music has been
shown to cause more blood flow to your brain, which can
improve your concentration skills and memory. Plus, listening to some music right before bedtime can help you
sleep better! So play on, young Nero!

In other words, music can have a profound effect on uplifting your spirit. Keep tapping into its power for your body,
mind, and spirit's own *good*. If you don't have a personal radio, CD, MP3, or tape player, consider getting one. To help
you select some invigorating new tunes, visit your local music store.

Besides shopping for healthier foods, supplements, and personal fitness needs, there are many other ways to activate your
mind, motivate your body, and uplift your spirit. Following is a
short list of subtle yet powerful changes you can make to your
environment that include little things I enjoy surrounding myself with such as stimulating music, aromatic candles, and inspirational books.

✳ **Candles.** Good lighting can soothe our senses. Bad lighting
can upset the atmosphere of any room. Because stress can
affect us negatively, adjust the lighting in your home and office so that it is appropriately crisp, yet not overly bright.
You may want to remove overly bright bulbs and replace

them with softer versions with less wattage. Or install dimmer switches, which cost about ten dollars. Lighting forever after? Priceless.

To help you unwind after a tough day buy a few aromatherapy candles to help create a more relaxing mood in your home. Aromatherapy is the art of using aromatic plants and essential oils for their alleged healing properties and dates back to the ancient Aztecs, Greeks, Romans, and Chinese. It can work aromatic wonders!

Go shopping and look around. You'll see everything from soothing bedtime lotions for kids featuring lavender and chamomile to plug-in jasmine-scented air fresheners. So go to a nearby mall or go on line and purchase aromatic products that can help transform a cold, sterile environment into a cozy, soothing space. You may enjoy an aromatherapy candle, a bowl of potpourri, bath beads, massage oils, or even a scented pillow.

Following is a short list of aromatherapy scents to choose from and how they may help:

* *Lavender* soothes, lifts moods, calms, and may help relieve tension.
* *Sandalwood* may help relieve stress, depression, exhaustion, and enhances sleep.
* *Jasmine* uplifts your spirit, helps you think more clearly, and relieves stress.
* *Rosemary* can calm your nerves, lessen stress, and enhance mental clarity.
* *Chamomile* has calming properties to help relieve stress and rock you to sleep.
* *Cinnamon* helps relieve stress and may improve your problem-solving abilities.
* *Lemon* may increase your ability to be accurate and make fewer mistakes.

✳ *Peppermint* invigorates the mind so you can remember things more clearly.

✳ **Books.** Books can transport you to faraway lands or help you discover practical ways to achieve a more fulfilling life. This book was designed as a launchpad for you to blast off onto your journey toward becoming a healthier, happier human being. After reading it, if you feel like boosting yourself to the next level of fitness or a deeper sense of personal happiness, search for books specific to your concerns. If you don't feel totally happy yet, for instance, look for titles that speak to a particular concern such as overcoming a dysfunctional childhood, or achieving spiritual happiness, or boosting self-esteem. There are dozens of great books out there to choose from that can help *you* . . . if you allow them.

Life is a journey, and it's okay to have fun along the way. Keep growing. Strive for more happiness. Continue to fine-tune your body into a beautiful instrument. In other words, find books that can help make your journey fantastic whenever you need them. Go on line if you are self-conscious or shy. Have the books discreetly mailed to your home. Choose to evolve into the happiest person you can possibly be. Why not?

Hints for Preparation

✳ Two words: Plan ahead. When you have healthy foods and ice-cold water within reach at all times, you will be much less likely to guzzle sodas and gobble junk.

✳ Begin searching for simple, easy-to-prepare, healthier meal ideas and recipes today. Ask friends and family for help. Buy magazines that feature family-friendly low-fat recipes. Visit a bookstore and buy a few cookbooks that look appealing to *you.* Go on line and type in the key words: "healthy recipes."

✳ Give yourself more time to prepare healthier dinners, sack lunches, and snacks for you and your family. How do you find more time? Consider simplifying your life. Many of us are doing way too much these days. Begin to eliminate those things that are not necessary to living a happier, more fulfilling life. Remember, expensive cars, clothing, and jewelry will not automatically make you happy . . . but a life filled with good food, fine beverages, love, laughter, friends, and family certainly can.

Time Savers

✳ Shop for all the groceries you will need for the entire week on Saturday or Sunday. Make a list of what you and your family will be eating for the week ahead. Planning ahead will make it possible to stop relying on fast foods and delivery pizza to fill in those ever-widening gaps in your nutritional repertoire.

✳ Begin cooking larger portions of appropriate dishes such as grilled skinless chicken breasts. Recycle them into sandwiches and pasta lunches and dinners later in the week. This can also help you take advantage of those larger "family packs" so often heavily discounted in price!

✳ Start serving more balanced and colorful meals. If making salads every single night is too time-consuming, toss a few prewashed and peeled vegetables with a drizzle of olive oil dressing on the side instead. The produce section is brimming with already prepared veggies these days. Take advantage of the healthful convenience.

✳ At home, chill and refrigerate foods as quickly as possible. Obviously, some items such as bananas and potatoes do not need refrigeration.

* Anytime you are preparing food wash your hands frequently with warm water and soap. You do not need to use antibacterial soaps.
* After you peel or cut into a fruit or vegetable refrigerate it right away. If leftover cut produce has been sitting at room temperature for over two hours, toss it out.
* Before eating fruit cut away any bruises first.
* Please note that most grocery stores do not wash produce before displaying it. So before eating produce always rinse with running water to reduce dirt and eliminate the toxic residue of pesticides. The best approach is to simply rinse fruits and vegetables with running water and then gently scrub them with a soft brush to loosen debris. You might also want to soak delicate items such as strawberries, which may have been sprayed many times with toxic pesticides, in cold or warm water first, for up to ten minutes, to help loosen dirt and toxins hiding in tiny crevices.
* If your place of work comes equipped with a fridge, take advantage of the convenience by keeping your own brown bag inside, stocked with a colorful variety of healthy choices like fruits, vegetables, prewashed legumes, and whole wheat products. From time to time, bring a few creative snack alternatives to munch on such as low-fat string cheese, push-up yogurts, grapes, carrot sticks, or oat bran pretzels. That way you'll be less apt to indulge in less-health-friendly items like those dripping in saturated fats, hydrogenated oils, and added sugars and salts.

Tips for Staying on Course

Ultimately, the decision to become healthier is yours. It isn't a magic bullet. It isn't some kind of extreme makeover surgery. It's a matter of deciding you want to do it. Then it's a matter of sticking with it for at least twenty-one days, allowing it to evolve naturally into your life. Remember, whether it's eating smaller meals more often, or making sure you get your five to nine servings of fruits and vegetables, or exercising for ten to twenty minutes at least three days a week, when you continue to do something for twenty-one days it will automatically and almost effortlessly become a new habit. After twenty-one days you will crave fresh fruits. You will yearn for the natural taste of vegetables. Your body will actually feel weird when you don't work out a little. It's that simple.

Everything you eat has an effect on your mind, body, and often your spirit. This is it, folks. You have one body. You have one mind. You have one totally unique spirit. Become more playful. Be nicer to friends, family, and even strangers. Be good to your *body*. Ponder this scenario for a moment: If you adopted an adorable puppy or a seasoned terrier from an animal shelter, would you feed your beloved new pet artery-clogging food with no nutritional value—for days, weeks, years on end? No, right? Then stop feeding your own precious body junk foods unfit for a dog!

Remind yourself that becoming more active will make you look better and help you feel more alive and energized. Exercising will firm up your physical assets, help you deal more effectively with stress, and reverse the signs of aging.

In the hours and days before you begin my 21-Day Guide, continue thinking about the many reasons why it's vital for *you* to make time for exercise a priority. Contemplate what it will take to get you to actually run, swim, dance, or hop on a bike. See what happens when you decide to get out of your car more often and walk. See what it would be like to stop relying on television to baby-sit you or your children so often. Consider the possibility of choosing to be more active *together*. Would time stand still if you . . . played catch in the backyard after supper? went bike riding on the weekends? Let your imagination run wild. Be creative. Find ways to become more active with friends, coworkers, and family that are fun for *you*.

Of course, to truly change for the longer, happier haul you need to find reasons that are important to *you*. If you are motivated by positive things to come, think about getting healthier as a way to ensure you live long enough to see your children or grandchildren get married. Or, think about how great it would feel to look sexier in a swimsuit this summer. Conversely, if you are more motivated by negative outcomes, think about what may really happen if you continue drinking to excess on a daily basis, or you allow your weight to continue climbing out of control.

Whatever your own personal reasons are for wanting to change your life for the better, make a list of what you expect to change over the next few weeks, months, and years. After you jot your reasons down on paper, set a firm date to begin my 21-day feel-good guide. Maybe you want to read the entire guide through first, and then set a date for your personal transformation to begin. Or perhaps you want to surprise yourself by reading and following along one day at a time. It's all up to you. Do it when it feels right for you. But don't keep putting it off indefinitely.

When you decide to go for the gold, tell a few close personal friends or family members that you are about to begin eating better and becoming more active. If they laugh, so what? Let their disapproval act as a catalyst for you to become more determined. If they approve, ask if they want to join along in the fun.

At all costs, continue taking responsibility for your own actions. You are in charge of your own nutritional destiny. You control the fate of how active you become. Your happiness and sex appeal are in your hands. If you work well with a carrot dangling before you, decide now how you will reward yourself upon completion of my guide. Maybe you'll decide to treat yourself to a fabulous salon makeover or splurge on a weekend of camping in the woods. Life is full of choices; make more of them good . . . for *you*.

Getting Ready to Jamba®!

Have you ever watched at a playground as children ran, screamed, and jumped to their hearts' content? They weren't worried about how many calories they ingested for lunch. They weren't thinking about fitness. They were simply having fun. Well, it's the essence of that same carefree spirit and the belief that inside all of us is a joyful child just waiting to break free from bad habits which is the heart of what brings forty million happy customers to Jamba each year and the soul of my 21-day fun-loving field guide.

In my opinion, no matter how well we hide it, deep inside each and every one of us lives a joyful, active child just waiting to come outside and play. Naturally, eating healthier foods and getting more exercise are part of the equation, but there is so much more to it than that. I know from experience that no matter which bad habits are personally holding *you* back—whether it's half a pack of cigarettes a day or a year without exercise—when you are truly ready for a big change . . .

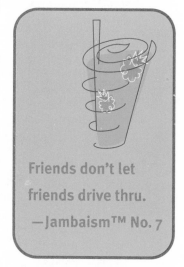

Friends don't let friends drive thru.

—Jambaism™ No. 7

when you really want to feel better for the long haul . . . when you decide it's time to stop buying the next bigger dress or pant size . . . that's when you'll know it's time to immerse yourself in the celebration of life!

I know because I've been on both sides of the fence. I've busted my buns at work and ignored working out. I've eaten fatty foods and gotten out of shape. I've also gone for weeks drinking healthful smoothies and enjoying a colorful diet rich in fruits, vegetables, legumes, whole-wheat grains, and fish. I've worked out properly for months and effectively competed in triathlons. I know what poor lifestyle choices feel like (rotten) and I know what good ones feel like (fantastic!) because I've experienced both. I have faith that when you begin experiencing the joys of healthier living you will love them too!

Once you begin the 21-day guide and hopefully follow it into the months and years to come, if you slip up and splurge on a high-fat breakfast, don't beat yourself up or throw in the towel; simply average it out later with a piece of fruit and a low-fat lunch. When you eat more than your daily recommended 6 ounces of meat, choose not to eat any meat for the rest of the day. Have a big colorful salad, a rice and bean burrito with spicy salsa, or a tasty plate of steamed veggies instead. If your workday consists of virtually no physical activity, choose to balance out your day with a morning or evening walk, jog, or swim. In other words, keep striving for balance and within time, a healthier, happier, sexier new you will replace the old one.

Within the first few days and weeks you may feel better. You may have more energy. You may look better. You may even lose weight, add muscle mass, and sleep like an angel. Your brain may work better. You may naturally feel more refreshed at work and you might be able to concentrate better. You may even feel less anxious or depressed. And, even though it's impossible to see, you may be reducing your risk of many diseases, including heart disease, high blood pressure, and strokes.

So, are you ready to Jamba?! To help you prepare for what could possibly be the most exciting, life-changing experience of your life, try the following: As you lie in bed tonight before falling asleep, think back to a time when you enjoyed running, jumping, or swimming. Remember what it felt like when you were more active and perhaps had fewer vices. Think about some long-forgotten, yet totally fun activities that you might enjoy again . . . like riding a bike in the countryside, swimming in a crystal blue lake, or skiing down a majestic mountain. Dream about the possibilities of living a cleaner, healthier, happier life. . . .

Chapter 4

A 21-Day Smoothie and Juice Guide

Week 1

Whether it's a short trip or a long one, every voyage begins with the first step. Often the first step for any type of change seems the most difficult, but as soon as you start moving toward your goal of becoming a little healthier, your journey will become easier and easier. As we mentioned, it takes twenty-one days to integrate a new habit into your lifestyle. With that in mind I've created a guide that helps you make that first step, and the twenty-one days that follow, as easy and pleasurable as possible.

Each day includes at least one easy-to-make smoothie or juice option that targets a specific need or body part that may need some fine-tuning. After all, who

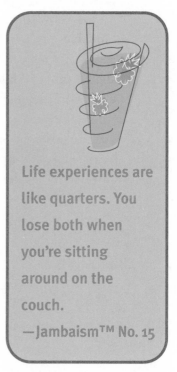

Life experiences are like quarters. You lose both when you're sitting around on the couch.
—Jambaism™ No. 15

doesn't want youthful-looking skin, a brain that functions at maximum capacity, or simply more energy? Each day also features a fun way to get your body moving—such as going for a quick walk during your lunch break or enrolling in a power yoga class on the weekends—and includes a de-stressing, nurturing thing you can do for yourself and sometimes others.

In addition, during this life-changing journey I'll help you integrate other healthy habits into your life, such as drinking lots of water, getting your five to nine servings of fruits and vegetables, eating more whole grains and legumes, controlling your intake of saturated fats, and getting plenty of rest and exercise. I'll teach you the difference between aerobic and anaerobic exercises as well as how and why each one can make a big difference in your overall well-being. Did you know, for instance, that being more active can improve your sex life, making it more pleasurable by increasing vital blood flow to sexual organs? Did you know that exercise boosts important chemicals in your brain that can increase your sense of self-esteem, boost your level of creativity, and make you feel really good—so good it is called a runner's high? I'll talk about why researchers now believe it's important for you to choose to eat five to six smaller meals a day rather than three big ones and why you should never intentionally starve yourself to lose weight because doing so can actually help you store more fat. That's my plan in a nutshell. These simple, small changes will painlessly add up to being more fit!

Day 1—Saturday: Let your 21-day journey begin!

Today is the perfect day to treat your body to the detoxifying elements of a satisfying fresh fruit smoothie, a nice long walk to clear your thoughts, and committing to making just a couple changes that will leave you feeling cleansed, relaxed, and less bogged down. To follow is a delicious idea for a nutritious, detoxifying smoothie along with a few suggestions of things to do today as well as how to plan for the week ahead.

Speaking of detoxifying, in chapter 1 you learned that *oxidation* is the process that turns the inside of an apple brown after it's been cut into. Oxidation also wreaks havoc on our health in basically the same way. Remember that the *free radicals* in our systems cause toxic damage to our cells that can lead to numerous diseases including bone weakening and rapid aging.

To ensure that your body and immune system get into and stay in good working order, a mini detox is in order. Don't worry, when I use the term *detox* I'm not talking about an odd colon-cleansing ritual or burning a bushel of sage to rid your home of evil spirits. I'm talking about spending some quality time in the great outdoors breathing fresh air and choosing to eat fewer overprocessed foods while enjoying a few more fruits and vegetables—

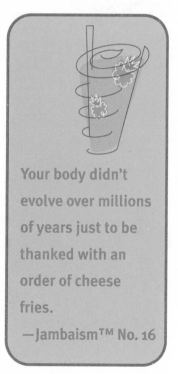

Your body didn't evolve over millions of years just to be thanked with an order of cheese fries.

—Jambaism™ No. 16

Nature's powerhouse of detoxifying antioxidants, phytochemicals, and vitamins!

Smoothie choice: Orange Oomph™

During the course of our multitasking, multilayered, modern lifetimes, we have all been exposed to an assortment of over-processed foods, air pollution, cigarette smoke, drugs, alcohol, and hundreds of other things that may be considered toxic, 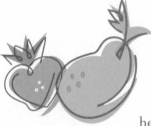 which means our systems may be teeming with damaging oxidants and free radicals. Mother Nature has provided us with a fruit-and-vegetable-powered crew for our internal toxic waste cleanup and disposal called phytochemicals—plant-derived components that help promote good health because of their antioxidant power, anti-inflammatory strength, and the way they help our bodies' natural ability to detoxify.

Begin the day with a vitamin-rich, fiber-intensive Orange Oomph Smoothie. (See recipe on page 186.) Besides the well-known power of OJ, new research at Tufts University in Boston shows that one cup of strawberries, which you'll find in the Orange Oomph recipe, contains a wide variety of phytochemicals, including anthocyanins (the pigment that gives the berries their red color while protecting them from being damaged by too much sun), ellagic and caffeic acid (two phytochemicals that have been shown to prevent tumors), as well as over 140 percent of your daily value of vitamin C, and many other vitamins and minerals.

Blueberries are powerful free-radical fighters as they contain more than a dozen important vitamins and minerals, plus nearly 100 detoxifying, disease-fighting phytochemicals including beta-carotene (a natural immune booster)—not to mention a storehouse of antioxidant and potent anti-inflammatory compounds.

Nutrition

* Did you know that you could probably survive for about thirty days without food but you probably wouldn't make it one full week without water? Water does all sorts of beneficial things for your body including helping to regulate your temperature and lubricating your joints. Water also helps carry nutrients through your body and *flush out toxins.* Try to drink at least eight glasses of water over the course of the day. A glass of water is 8 ounces. An easy way to do this is to buy one liter of bottled water. Drink that bottle, fill it up again and when you finish the second one you've fulfilled your daily water requirement.

* Other foods containing water include: lettuce at 96 percent, watermelon at 93 percent, broccoli at 91 percent, raw carrots at 88 percent, raw apples at 85 percent, grapes at 82 percent, and bananas at 76 percent. As you can see, eating lots of fresh fruits and veggies can help you get all the water your body needs! So strive to get your five to nine servings of fruits and veggies every day.

* Try to eat five small meals a day instead of three big ones, and keep mixing and matching different colored fruits and vegetables to complement every meal. Because you started the day with an Orange Oomph Smoothie, have a golden delicious apple as a snack later in the day with a small handful of almonds. For dinner, choose an assortment of green and yellow vegetables as side dishes. Later, have a small bowl of grapes or peach slices with a cup of low-fat yogurt.

Activity

Today is Saturday so you probably have some time to walk around, to stop and smell the flowers, and generally pay more attention to the things around you. Find some time during the day simply to walk around your neighborhood, or in nature. Walk for as long as you want, but today try to do it for at least ten minutes. Walk at whatever speed feels right for you. This isn't a race. Walking is considered one of the most effective and safest forms of aerobic exercise you can do. An aerobic exercise is simply one that makes your heart and lungs work a little bit harder to get more vital oxygen to your muscles. Plus, walking is one of the easiest and most pleasurable things you can do. It's good for your body; it helps control body fat, tones muscles, aids in your body's natural detoxifying system by cleaning out your liver and pancreas, and it also clears your head.

It's best to start out walking slowly, but when you're ready to walk at a quicker pace, consider the fact that researchers at California State University have found that merely ten minutes of brisk walking can boost your mood and your energy level for up to two hours afterward. Go for a walk alone or with friends and see how much fun you can have.

Mind/Body/Spirit

A great way to continue with your detox is to draw yourself a nice relaxing hot bath. While you're running the water, pour in one or two cups of Epsom salts. Epsom salts are named for the natural waters of Epsom, England, where they have been enjoyed for their healing properties since Shakespeare's day. Epsom salts, a mineral known to scientists as magnesium sulfate, can help draw impurities out of your system.

Turn out the lights and light a soothing aromatherapy candle. I like the soothing aromatic scent of lavender and orange blossoms. Sink into the detoxifying Epsom salt tub for twenty minutes or so. The hot water will help relax you. When you come out, you'll feel like a new person. See, doing good things for yourself also feels good.

(FYI: Epsom salts can be used by most people on a daily basis; however, do not use them if you have high blood pressure or a kidney condition.)

Day 2—Sunday
Smoothie choice: Raspberry Royale™

Sunday is typically known as the day when we can truly relax, reflect, and rejuvenate our minds, bodies, and spirits. Today is especially dedicated to your rejuvenation—with the nutritional focus on reinvigorating the vitality of your skin. Did you know that skin is actually the largest organ in your body? It not only helps protect you from environmental elements like sun and wind but it's also an important organ to help you eliminate toxins. Every month your skin cells renew themselves. To jump-start the renewal process, wake up and blend yourself one of my specially formulated Raspberry Royale Smoothies. (See recipe on page 199.)

Nutrition

* Besides the important benefits of water you learned about yesterday, drinking ample fluids or eating plenty of fruits and vegetables also helps rejuvenate the appearance of your skin because, as we mentioned, it helps eliminate toxins. In fact, most doctors agree that drinking plenty of water may be the most important thing you can do to have healthy-looking skin. Instead of a fifth or sixth cup of coffee that can dry out your skin because of its diuretic effects, reach for another glass of water.
* Consider having a leafy vegetable or two for lunch or dinner. Leafy greens are high in vitamin A, which is also terrific for your skin's health. Think: spinach, dark green leafy lettuce, cabbage, the exotic Swiss chard, watercress, or kale.
* Other antioxidants found naturally in fruits like beta-carotene and vitamin C are also great for youthful-looking skin. So enjoy a refreshing splash of OJ, an ice-cold glass of

cranberry juice, or a revitalizing tropical nectar like mango or papaya juice.

Activity

Whether it's the ocean, a nearby lakeshore, or an indoor swimming pool, get yourself to a body of water today and go for a short swim. Swimming is another fantastic aerobic activity that people of all ages can enjoy. The more aerobic activities you introduce into your life, the more energy you will have. If you have kids, take them with you and simply splash around or play a rousing game of Marco Polo.

Marco Polo can be played with three or more people. To start, one person is designated "it." Then he closes his eyes, goes under water, and quickly counts to twenty while the others swim away. After counting to twenty, the one designated it pops up and, keeping his eyes closed, pursues the others by touch. To locate the others, he calls out "Marco," to which they must respond "Polo," and the chase is on. The game continues— "Marco"—"Polo"—"Marco"—"Polo"—until one of the others is caught and then he becomes it. Repeat until happily exhausted.

If you don't enjoy swimming, stroll around the perimeter of the pool or along the shore. The longer you enjoy any activity, the more beneficial it will be for your overall health, happiness, and sex appeal. Just try to be active for at least ten minutes. While walking or resting after swimming, allow your mind to clear and reflect.

Mind/Body/Spirit

During the day, reconfirm your commitment to becoming a healthier you. What do you really want to achieve during this 21-Day Plan? Do you simply want to have a better understanding of the basics of nutrition and how fruits and vegetables can help? Do you want help in accepting your body? Do you need a few simple tips to help you lose weight? Would you like to take control of your life? Define what it is you really want and then set your own, very personal, yet realistic goals. Write your promise down on paper. Hang it where it's visible—perhaps on the bathroom mirror or the refrigerator—or fold it up and put it in your wallet or purse. If you would like support, call a friend or family member and ask him or her to join you on your quest.

Day 3—Monday
Smoothie choice: Apricot Affinity™

Ye Olde Dreaded Monday has arrived—but this morning, this Monday morning, of this very special week is destined to be different. You are on a brand-new voyage to change your life, and what better way to do that than to start off your day in a *good mood?* There can be no denying that what you eat and drink affects your mood. Often we self-medicate with foods and drinks that change our brain chemistry to make us feel instantly better—things like caffeinated beverages, sweets, and treats. That's because the chemicals found in sugar and caffeine can give our brains an instant rush of pleasure.

Our moods can also be positively affected by many other carbohydrate-rich foods that we eat, especially those that increase a chemical transmitter in our brains called serotonin. Many antidepressants work to increase levels of serotonin. When you don't have enough of it, you can get depressed. That's why many people who feel tired, cranky, or depressed first turn to sugar. Sugar gives us relief—a buzz, if you will. The trouble is that refined sugar is a *simple* carbohydrate that will soon wear off leaving you less alert and less energetic than you started. A *complex* carbohydrate, on the other hand, found in foods like fruits, whole-grain cereals, and oatmeal takes longer to move through your system so you have energy that lasts longer. That's why I recommend turning to a fruit-and-fiber-filled, complex-carbohydrate-rich smoothie like the Apricot Affinity, to boost your mood. (See recipe on page 166.)

Nutrition

* Foods such as oat bran, tuna, Brazil nuts, and sunflower seeds are high in selenium. Selenium has been proven to improve moods. Bring a small bag of Brazil nuts or sunflower seeds to work to snack on as part of your new five-smaller-meals-a-day plan.

* To maintain a good mood throughout the afternoon—when most of us feel sluggish—have an energizing spinach salad for lunch. Spinach and other leafy green vegetables are loaded with folic acid (which is a B vitamin). Low levels of folic acid have been proven by scientists to be a major contributor to depression.

* Tonight enjoy a broiled-fish dinner (farm-raised trout or salmon are terrific choices), then later as a mini-meal munch on a golden delicious apple, an orange, or a juicy peach.

Activity

Go for a walk during your lunch hour, even if it's just around your work neighborhood or office building. If you have the time, drive to a nearby park or waterfront area and enjoy a nice walk courtesy of Mother Nature. You'll feel so refreshed when you get back to work that the afternoon will fly by.

Mind/Body/Spirit

The beauty of Mother Nature can have a profound effect on your inner sense of well-being. While you're out and about in this peaceful surrounding, enjoying the sunshine (with some sunscreen and sunglasses on to protect your skin and eyes from aging too quickly), breathing the fresh air, take a few moments to contemplate joy and a job well done so far. You made it through three days!

Day 4—Tuesday
Juice choice: Carrot Creation™

Instead of coffee this morning, try switching to a cup of cancer-fighting green or black tea. Many studies have shown that tea can help protect your arteries, fight infections and cavities, and block various types of cancer from striking. After a delightful cup, do something nice for your eyes by mixing up an incredible eye-opening, vision-enhancing Carrot Creation. (See recipe on page 211.)

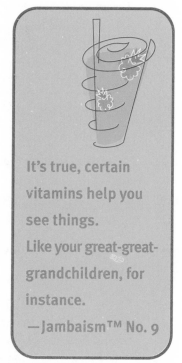

Nutrition

It's true, certain vitamins help you see things.

Like your great-great-grandchildren, for instance.

—Jambaism™ No. 9

* Bring a bag of already prepared veggies with you to work. Snack on them over the course of the day. Studies show that when you fill up on nutritious fruits and veggies you are less likely to reach for junk foods. Plus, carrots are full of the orange pigment known as beta-carotene. Besides being a powerful antioxidant, beta-carotene is a major source of vitamin A, which is important for vision.

* Another great antioxidant for your eyes is lutein. Lutein can be found in all sorts of vegetables, namely, spinach, red peppers, romaine lettuce, kale, and broccoli. Today for lunch or tonight for dinner do your eyes another favor and have a colorful salad featuring any or all of the veggies mentioned above you. Top it with an olive oil– or canola oil–based vinaigrette—the only oily way to go.

* Keep drinking your eight glasses of water during the day.

Snacking on unhealthful foods has nearly doubled in the last decade. How do so many of us get suckered into it? Hmm, 70 percent of food advertising is for conveniently packaged candies, soft drinks, alcoholic beverages, and snacks. But guess how much is spent on advertising all other healthier foods such as fruits and vegetables? A minuscule 2 percent!

Activity

Can you imagine life without music? Today turn up your stereo and while you are listening to your all-time favorite music—whether it's slow, fast, or hard rock—dance, dance, and dance some more. If you consider yourself to be a terrible dancer, shut the drapes or pull the blinds and dance as if no one is watching—because no one is! Just enjoy yourself without any inhibitions.

You may also find that going for a walk yesterday during lunch felt so good that you want to do it again. Today set your walk to music by putting on your headphones and taking off around the block or to a nearby park at a slightly quicker pace. By the time you get back to the office, your face will probably have a new glow and you'll be eager to tell anyone interested about your healthy new progress.

Mind/Body/Spirit

Numerous studies have shown that support and encouragement from friends, family, and coworkers can go a long way toward helping us achieve our goals. Today, confide in people whom you trust about your quest to become a little healthier. Ask a friend if he or she has any delicious fruit- or vegetable-filled recipes to share with you or enlist coworkers to go on lunchtime walks with you. If someone you already know or a new person you meet during the day appears to be in particularly good shape, inquire about how he or she got so fit.

This afternoon or evening when you get home from work, rather than eating the first thing you see in the fridge or grabbing a candy bar, try mixing up a sweet and tangy Tropical Tease Smoothie to quench your thirst and sweet tooth. (See recipe on page 207.) If you're really counting calories, try a Carrot Apple Squeeze instead. (See recipe on page 210.)

Day 5—Wednesday
Smoothie choice: Pomegranate Pom-Poms™

Because you're probably already feeling a lot better than you did last week, congratulate yourself by having a big bowl of oatmeal or other oat-based cereal and a bowl of fresh (or recently thawed) berries for breakfast. Eaten regularly, oats can help lower bad (LDL) cholesterol by up to 10 percent in some people. Oats can also help stabilize blood sugar levels, which means your energy levels will remain more constant throughout the day. Besides being a complex carbohydrate, oats contain psychoactive compounds that may help you resist cigarette cravings. Plus, oats have antidepressant powers. To complement this amazing yet simple breakfast, make your own Pomegranate Pom-Poms Smoothie. (See recipe on page 197.)

While you are slowly sipping this satisfying treat, consider the additional fact that this smoothie choice can help your body keep growing properly because it helps maintain vital functions like cell repair and it has healthy levels of vitamin B_6 that will help you fight fatigue, anxiety, and muscle pain. B_6 is also important for women because it helps hormone balance and can lessen the effects of water retention, which can lead to soreness in the breasts and even emotional tension. Plus, this drink is also high in calcium and phosphorus needed for strong bones and teeth.

Nutrition

✳ Most of us have heard that vitamin D is important for bone strength, and now research shows that other minerals can help, too, namely *potassium* and *magnesium*. Because bananas, oranges, and cantaloupes are great sources of *potassium* bring one, two, or all three with you to work today and enjoy!

✳ Terrific sources of the mineral *magnesium* for strong bones include dark breads, peanut butter, chicken, and fish. For lunch or dinner, enjoy a healthy filet of baked salmon or grilled chicken without the fatty skin. As a side dish indulge in a big plate of your favorite steamed or fresh vegetables and a little brown rice.

✳ Keep drinking plenty of fluids such as water and consider having a glass of tomato, vegetable, or carrot juice at some point during the day.

Activity

Sometimes the biggest barrier to our becoming more active is a perceived lack of time. But in the ten minutes it takes to talk to 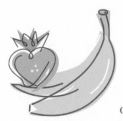 a friend on your cell phone or brush and floss your teeth, you could be boosting your cardiovascular endurance, building muscle, and increasing flexibility. So today, forget about the notion that you can't get into shape unless you go to a gym or a track for an hour. Instead sneak in a brief workout or two—something active for just ten minutes, two or three times if you like. Take your pick from the following activities: go for a walk, climb stairs, or march in place.

Mind/Body/Spirit

Have you ever noticed how wonderful it feels to give something to another person? I'm talking about giving someone something for no reason at all. The side effect of giving to others is personal joy. Today go out of your way to be giving to as many people as you can. For instance: Bring a flower to your office assistant. Give a coworker a quick pat on the back for a job well done. Send a note to a friend even if it's brief, or leave a message of love for a family member or lover. Compliment a stranger on her colorful blouse or his radiant smile.

Day 6—Thursday
Smoothie choice: Aloha Pineapple™

All right, it's Thursday—which means there's only one more whole day until the weekend. To help you fantasize about the fun you're going to have, wake up a few minutes early and sail into a freshly made Aloha Pineapple Smoothie, which is also available at Jamba stores. (See recipe on page 161.) Not only is this drink tasty; it's also high in vitamin C, calcium, and manganese, so your bones won't get brittle and you will have less trouble with your teeth. This smoothie is also a great source of fiber for digestive health, plus iron for oxygen flow in the blood to promote high levels of much needed energy!

Nutrition

* As a midmorning mini-meal have a cup of low-fat cottage cheese, an apple, and a small handful of whole-wheat pretzels.
* Instead of eating another fast-food hamburger and french fries for lunch, have a turkey sandwich on whole-wheat

bread. On the side have a big salad or as many cooked vegetables as you want.

* Snack on fresh fruit and a few whole-wheat crackers in the afternoon.
* Have a baked apple or a poached pear as a side dish at dinnertime. Keep yourself hydrated with plenty of fluids including ice cold water.

Activity

During your lunch break, call a good friend on your cell phone or invite a group of friendly coworkers for a brisk ten- to twenty-minute walk and concentrate on having a few laughs. Laughing is good for your stomach muscles and great for your state of mind!

Mind/Body/Spirit

Socializing with friends, having some laughs, and forgetting your troubles for a while is a great way to relax and bring pleasure into your life. Too often in our hectic day-to-day lives and obligations we forget to connect with the people we love. It's Thursday, so there is still time to plan for a group of friends and/or family members to get together over the weekend. Do something fun and different like bowling or roller-skating, both of which are a lot healthier than simply going clothes shopping or watching sports on TV; it's active and is sure to be a crowd pleaser. You'll feel great knowing you brought everyone together and that you got everyone, including yourself, moving.

Day 7—TGIF!

Smoothie choice: Giddy Guava™

You've almost made it through an entire week of eating better and being a little more active. Don't you feel a whole lot better?

Because you've been so good this week, here are a couple of smoothie choices you can create and enjoy to celebrate the end of your first healthier week—and the beginning of a lifetime of better living:

* Cantaloupe Caress™ (See recipe on page 169.)
* Cherish the Cherries™ (See recipe on page 170.)

Or maybe you'd like to celebrate by going Giddy Guava! That's right, because you have successfully completed your first full week of healthier living, wake up and smell the mangoes inside my Giddy Guava Smoothie. (See recipe on page 174.)

Nutrition

* Today, give yourself a break. Have something sinful for lunch or dinner. Sure, you can still go for a brisk walk before, during, or after work if you want and you can keep squeezing in a piece of fruit or two.
* If you want to continue being really good, go easy on your meat portions, skip overindulging in foods high in saturated fats like french fries, and avoid sugary, empty-calorie beverages like soda.
* Remember to drink plenty of fluids, especially water.

Activity

It's Friday night—so get your significant other and a good friend or two together and go out dancing. Not every dance club is a rowdy singles scene, so ask around and find a place where you'll feel comfortable letting loose. If going out on the town isn't your cup of tea, get everyone together at your place for a healthy potluck dinner. Ask each guest to bring their favorite healthy dish and a CD they enjoy dancing to. After dinner crank up the music and dance. Make sure to get a good night's sleep though, because next week you will be given even more little things to think about and fun activities to do—to make you healthier, happier, and sexier with almost no sacrificing or extra effort!

Mind/Body/Spirit

Before you go out dancing or your friends arrive for dinner, take a few minutes to write some thoughts down in a journal. How did the small habit changes you made during the past week make you feel—did you notice a difference in your energy levels? Did that post-lunch fatigue magically disappear? Were you more energized to get up in the morning? Did you feel like you were sleeping better? Maybe that heartburn or acid stomach you've become so used to wasn't there anymore? Did you feel more relaxed, a little happier? Did a rosy glow return to your skin? Maybe you had some real fun for the first time in a long time. Think about what really made you feel better this past week and reinforce your commitment to stay on the plan for week number two. Tomorrow is going to be chock-full of fun things to do and tasty, healthier things to eat!

Week 2—
The Fun Continues

Congratulations on making it through your first full week of healthier living. Week two is important because here you will learn the bulk of information needed to continue your journey long after these first twenty-one days are over. Don't worry about being bombarded with too much info or too many technical terms. I will keep everything simple so at each step of the way, you will continue having fun.

As for what's ahead nutritionally, today our focus will center on learning about which fats are the best and worst for your body. Sunday I'll talk about sugar. Starting with Monday and continuing through Friday, each day we will explore some amazing facts about the five major food groups. On Monday it's proteins—including meats, bean, and nuts. Tuesday it's dairy and soy. Wednesday we'll explore more fascinating things about the power of fruits. Thursday is dedicated to vegetables. And Friday you'll learn about whole-grain breads, cereals, and pastas.

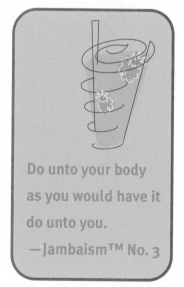

Do unto your body as you would have it do unto you.
—Jambaism™ No. 3

This week I will also show you how to sneak about ten to twenty more minutes of activity into your day. Not only will you continue doing aerobic—or "with oxygen"—exercises, the kind that get your heart to beat a little faster, but you will also be exposed to some anaerobic exercise. Technically speaking, *anaerobic* means "without oxygen." Anaerobic activities are those in which your body uses oxygen more quickly than your body can supply it. Lifting weights is the most common example of an anaerobic exercise. Other examples include baseball and some forms of yoga. They help you build muscle strength and endurance—and every multitasking Tom, Dick, and harried soccer mom knows how important it is to have long-lasting strength and endurance!

If you have problems with your back, bones, or joints, a few less stressful strength-training activities include: isometric exercises using your own body for resistance, aquatic workouts using the resistance of water to build strength, and Pilates, a ballet-derived workout that will strengthen your abs and lower back and tighten your derrière.

Again, each day continue striving toward eating about five smaller meals, mixing up your five to nine servings of colorful fruits and veggies, and switching to whole-grain products. Slow down on snack foods with saturated fats and hydrogenated oils, and avoid drinking too much alcohol. And, keep striving for about eight hours of sleep every night! Otherwise, let's get to it. It's time to take a few more baby steps toward better health.

Day 8—Saturday
Smoothie choice: **Apple Kiwi Kosmo™**

Today is the beginning of your second week toward becoming a healthier, happier, sexier you! It's also a great day to get a few things done and have some fun. Get off to an energizing start by popping into a Jamba Juice store, if one is handy, and ordering an Apple Kiwi Kosmo Smoothie, or sleep in late and make your own at home. (See recipe on page 164.) In any event, don't wait too long upon waking to eat or drink something nutritious. You need fuel for energy. Remember, when you don't eat for prolonged periods of time your body stores energy as fat! Keep striving to eat five or six light meals a day, especially if you are trying to keep your weight under control.

Speaking of weight-controlling tips, did you also know that it isn't the fat we eat that makes us pack on the pounds? Generally, it's that we eat too many calories and don't burn them off. Sure, ounce for ounce fat actually weights more than other compounds in food. In fact, one gram of fat equals nine calories, whereas a gram of protein or carbohydrate only has four. However, if you remember from chapter 2, "Power Foods, Power Fruits, and Jamba Boosts!," the important thing to note is that *not all fats are bad.* In fact, certain oils and essential fatty acids are valuable keys to superior health.

In your body, energy is stored mostly as fat. Fat *provides* energy. Fat also acts as a carrier for many vitamins such as A, D, E, and K, helping them to become absorbed into your system. Your internal organs need fat for insulation. And because your body doesn't make certain fats on its own—essential fatty acids, to be more precise—*you need to get fats from your diet.*

To feel confident about which fats are the best ones for you, let me break down fats into their basic categories of good versus bad:

Good

* **Monounsaturated fats** usually come from plants and include: canola and olive oils, canola margarine, peanuts, and avocados.
* **Polyunsaturated fats** come from fish and some vegetable oils. This category is divided into two groups: omega-3 and omega-6. Omega-3 (alpha-linolenic) oil can be found mainly in canola oil, soybean oil, and fish. Omega-6 (linoleic) oil can be found mostly in safflower, sunflower, and corn oils.

These fats are wonderful to your body because they help you fight heart disease and may even prevent cancer and diabetes.

Plus, eating fish—especially tuna, salmon, and sardines—that contain the amazing omega-3 fatty acids may help reduce the risk of heart attacks and protect your entire cardiovascular system. Linseed and flax oil also contain lots of omega-3s!

Bad

* **Saturated fats** are from animal foods like meats, cheeses, and milk.
* **Trans-fatty acids** are a by-product of hydrogenation.

What's wrong with choosing too many saturated fats? *Saturated fats* put you at greater risk for health hazards like heart attacks and disease and raise bad cholesterol levels. So choose to limit your saturated-fat intake to less than 20 grams a day, about 10 percent of your total daily calories, or about a third of your overall fat intake.

Trans-fatty acids are formed through a process called hydrogenation, which extends the shelf-life of products and helps them stay crunchy. Scientifically speaking, hydrogenation transforms oils into a liquid or a solid form at room temperature, by rearranging the hydrogen atoms. This process is the one that is used to create "hydrogenated and partially hydrogenated vegetable oils." Avoid these whenever possible, which I know can be tough because they are found in many processed snack foods.

Personally, it's none of my business whether you are big, small, large, or tall. Happiness, integrity, intelligence, and compassion come from within. Those are the kinds of traits that are important. However, obesity is clearly bad for your health and it can have profoundly negative effects on your level of happiness. If you are having trouble slimming down on your own, see a doctor; you may need medication.

The American Obesity Association states that obesity:

✳ Increases the risk of illness from almost thirty serious medical conditions, and it's associated with increases in deaths from all causes.

✳ Can lead to earlier onset of obesity-related diseases, such as type II diabetes, which is now being reported in children and adolescents with obesity more often.

✳ Places you at higher risk for impaired mobility.

✳ Can lead to social stigmatization and discrimination in employment and academic situations.

Most doctors now believe that heredity plays a key role in determining whether or not a person will become obese. In addition, a stressful life situation such as the death of a loved one, job loss, or even a change in medication can dramatically increase your risk for becoming obese. In any case, obesity has less to do with your willpower and more to do with a problem with your brain chemistry.

In essence, your brain acts like your body's command center, controlling everything from your mood to your appetite. If you constantly crave sweets or salty or fatty foods or are hungry all the time, you may have a glitch in your hunger switch. If you have tried every diet known to mankind and nothing works or you eat like a bird and never lose weight, your brain may have switched your body into a terminal starvation mode, storing most of its energy as fat. If any of these scenarios apply to you, you may have an imbalance of brain chemicals called neurotransmitters. Neurotransmitters basically pass messages from one area of your brain to another. Your brain needs these transmitters because its cells do not touch one another.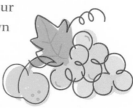

Transmitters such as norepinephrine give you energy and help you control hunger. Without enough norepinephrine you may feel depressed, exhausted, and constantly hungry. If you recall, serotonin is a neurotransmitter than can lift your mood and suppress your appetite. Serotonin levels also have an effect on anxiety, arousal, aggression, and even the way you think. Dopamine sends pleasurable messages from one cell in your brain to another. And dopamine not only helps you feel pleasure but also makes you want to seek out more of it! Alcohol, cigarettes, and illegal street drugs can increase dopamine levels, and that's why they are so addictive. For more information, ask your doctor about medications or natural supplements that may help. I also recommend reading, *Turn Off the Hunger Switch Naturally*, by Paul Rivas, M.D.

If obesity is not a common family trait but you are uncertain whether you are actually overweight or obese, check with your doctor. If you've simply been gaining a little unwanted weight and want to decrease your size or prevent yourself from becoming obese, make a decision to balance the number of calories you get from foods and beverages with the amount of energy you use up through activities. Remember: Every extra pound of fat we carry with us contains 3,500 calories. To lose one pound of fat a week you simply need to burn 500 calories a day through exercising or eat 500 fewer calories of junk foods.

FACT FUNFASTFACT FUNFASTFACT FUNFASTFACT FUNFASTFACT
UNFASTFACT FUNFASTFACT FUNFASTFACT FUNFASTFACT FUNFA

Drop a few pounds for your children's sake. Why? Studies show that 80 percent of the kids born to overweight parents will become obese, whereas, only 14 percent of the children who have parents within normal ranges of weight will become obese.

One easy way to help you burn more calories without really trying is to eat five or six smaller more nutritious meals a day, as I've been advocating. When you eat, you increase your metabolic rate—the rate at which you burn energy. The body is programmed to *store energy as fat* when you eat fewer larger meals. When you graze lightly, you tend to *use stored fat as energy*. So eating smaller meals more often every day will make you more efficient at burning calories. Again, anytime you go for long periods without eating your brain tells your body that something is wrong and you go into starvation mode, in which your body saves everything it can in the form of fat.

Nutrition

* Today switch to salad dressings made with olive oil or canola oil. They are the best *for your body*. Don't go overboard. Calories can add up quickly. Even a healthy monounsaturated fat like olive oil still has 2 grams of saturated fat per tablespoonful, so use oil sparingly.
* As a suppertime side dish enjoy a baked sweet potato au natural, or a good old-fashioned Idaho spud. Instead of heaping on the butter, bacon bits, and sour cream, try topping it with a zesty salsa, low-fat yogurt, or low-fat sour cream.
* One easy way to eat your five to nine servings of fruits and veggies is to eat one naturally delicious and nutritious fruit or veggie with each of your five smaller meals today. A slice of honeydew melon, a banana, or a bowl of ripe strawberries is a sensational choice. A bag of carrots, a red bell pepper, a few celery stalks can complement any meal or snack as well.
* Do you want to drop a few pounds effortlessly? Consider this idea: If you replace a daily 16-ounce soda with a glass of water, you can lose twenty pounds in a year! So drink your eight glasses of water and slim down without even trying.

Activity

Let's concentrate on finding some fun ways to become a little more active that are also designed to help boost your resting metabolism so your body will burn calories quicker, even while you are sleeping! The best way to do that is through anaerobic activity. Remember, anaerobic exercise is something that uses oxygen more quickly than your body can supply it. Personally, I like training with weights in a gym and I have found that mornings work best for me. If weight lifting sounds like something you'd like to try or get back into, go for it. Buy a few light dumbbells at a sporting-goods store today. Or join a nearby gym and ask for instructions on how to use everything properly. If you can afford fifty to a hundred extra bucks, I really recommend hiring a personal trainer to help you get started, even if it's just for a few sessions.

For those of you who can't imagine lifting weights for whatever personal reasons you may have, visit a video store or library with a video section. Search for a few titles that sound fun *to you!* I can't tell you which videos will inspire you to become more active; only *you* can decide that. What I can tell you is to look for videos that feature some kind of strength-training exercises, ones that emphasize isometric exercises or calisthenics such as push-ups and abdominal crunches. Look for a title sounding something like *Power Yoga, Pilates,* or even *Kickboxing with Granny.* If possible, buy or rent at least three titles that sound interesting to *you.*

If you have kids and want to involve them in your activity, there are plenty of great titles to choose from with your own adorable Mini Mimi in mind. Try *Movin' & Groovin' Fitness for Kids, Tae Bo for Kids, Children's Pilates,* or something superfun like Sesame Street's *Elmosize!*

Sometime during the day—if you're like me, the earlier the better—put on some comfortable clothes, draw the blinds if you are self-conscious, and pop in a video. If you don't like the first one, eject and remove. If you don't like the second, try the third. When you find one that feels right for you, just sit back and watch for a while without moving a muscle. Soak it all in. The instructor will likely explain why he or she is doing each exercise and which area of the body it is helping. Watch carefully and try to commit to memory as many of the basic stretching, warm-up, and strength-training moves as possible. The strength-training exercises will be the slower, more deliberate moves like leg squats, push-ups, and isometric arm exercises. All these moves will be ones you can do on your own later in the week. Keep watching, and when the music has just the right beat for you and the mood begins to strike, follow along for at least ten to twenty minutes—more if you like. Don't overdo it, though. The old phrase "no pain, no gain" is a myth. Instead you should take it very slowly—especially if it's been a while since you were active. You don't want to get out of breath, start panting, or feel faint. If you do, stop and relax for a while! Roman statues were not built in a day.

Modern health experts recommend both aerobic *and* strength-building exercises because each has a different effect on your soon-to-be sexier body. Both are beneficial. If you only do one, you won't get the full benefits. No one is asking you to become an Olympic athlete overnight. Becoming fit is a slow process, but I know for a fact that it can also be a lot of fun. Ten minutes here and twenty minutes there add up. Before you know it, your spirits have been lifted. You feel more energetic. Your body becomes firmer. You look sexier.

In the days and weeks ahead keep figuring out ways to make becoming more active interesting for *you*. Stick with the ones you like for as long as you can. But remember: When you do something for twenty-one days, it will become a new healthy habit.

Mind/Body/Spirit

Researchers from the University of Kansas recently found out that women who start an exercise program and give up shortly afterward do so because their initial expectations are way too high. Don't let that happen to you. Think about which benefits are reasonable to expect by the time you have finished with these twenty-one days. Again, nothing I ask you to do for the remaining thirteen days will be enormously difficult; however, you must realize that the results you are just starting to experience are subtle. We all have certain gifts, certain body types. So relax. Don't beat yourself up for being a little out of shape. Keep making a little progress daily and you will continue to become fit.

Tonight, spend a few moments alone while you are taking a bath or showering and think about all the positive traits you have that make you special. Maybe you are good with children. Perhaps you are gentle with seniors. For whatever good qualities you have, give yourself a round of applause. Love yourself for who you are right now. You've been given one unique mind, body, and spirit that will last your lifetime. Decide that you want to continue making small changes to take care of it. You can't change everything or conquer all your problems in one fell swoop. But slowly and surely you can transform yourself into the healthiest, happiest, sexiest person *you* can possibly be. And I have confidence that you are worth it!

Day 9—Sunday
Smoothie choice: Pacific Passion™

Day nine—wow! Congratulate yourself on making it this far! Because it's Sunday, spend most of the day relaxing. And what better way to start the day than with a silky, smooth Pacific Passion Smoothie. (See recipe on page 189.) How can this delightful drink help you on your continuing quest for better health? It's low in fat and high in vitamins B_6 and B_3, which Mother Nature designed to support your nervous system and help your body convert food into energy. Plus, it's loaded with vitamin C to help your body resist stress, which we'll get into more in week three.

Yesterday we discussed the importance of choosing to use good oils like olive and canola. Today while resting we'll focus for a few minutes on gaining a little better understanding of why health professionals are always asking us to eat sweets sparingly.

One of the most obvious reasons we are asked to slow down on sweets is that most sugary products don't really make us feel full. Believe me, I know how easy it is to eat way too many sweets without giving it much thought. Other times we gobble up a bagful of sugar cookies or guzzle down a big soda when we are feeling overwhelmed or deeply stressed.

Another more serious problem for many involves an imbalance of blood sugar levels. After digestion, sugar and starches change into glucose—the simplest form of sugar—which is vital to body cells for energy and growth. Eating sugar causes your blood sugar level to rise quickly. To counteract, your pancreas—a long gland behind your stomach that secretes insulin into your bloodstream—starts making insulin. Insulin acts like a key that opens the door to cells and allows sugar or glucose to enter. After the sugar spikes upward, your blood sugar levels fall back down, only this time lower than where they started. You feel tired and run-down, so you may eat more sugar or drink another soda to pick you back up—inadvertently ingesting hundreds of nonnutritious calories.

Eating and drinking too many calories of simple sugars along with not getting enough exercise has been linked to the increasing development of adult-onset diabetes. In fact, according to doctors at the Centers for Disease Control in Atlanta, 33 percent of the children born in the year 2000 will develop diabetes. For Hispanic and black kids, it's between 40 and 50 percent. Another sad fact is that two out of every three people with diabetes will develop heart disease, while many others may go blind, experience kidney failure, and/or need amputations.

So what is diabetes exactly? Diabetes is a disorder where the body can't make proper use of carbohydrates—especially those found in sugar and starches.

* **Type I diabetes** is usually found in children and young adults. It occurs when one's pancreas produces little or no insulin. My twin sister suffers from this type. She spends a lot of time every day monitoring her blood sugar levels and what she eats. She also has to wear a pump that provides her with insulin. It is not fun.

* **Type II diabetes** or adult-onset diabetes, happens to people usually as adults, especially the overweight and inactive. This type of diabetes is showing up in younger people, even kids, more often nowadays. Many experts believe it's because of poor diets, sugar overload, and lack of exercise. Type II diabetes can be treated and prevented by eating a healthier diet and by getting plenty of exercise—exactly what you are doing right now!

For more information on preventing and controlling both types of diabetes, check out the American Diabetes Association's website, www.diabetes.org.

Nutrition

* Choose to eat apples, bananas, or oranges as snacks today rather than simply drinking a glass of juice or soda. Sure, juice is better than a soft drink—but the fiber in fruits will

help keep your sugar levels more stable and help you maintain energy longer. So keep those five to nine servings of fruits and vegetables coming!

❊ Instead of indulging every sweet tooth you have with too many calories, consider switching to a piece of fruit, sugar-free gum, or a frozen juice bar.

❊ After dinner, have a bowl of fresh (or thawed) berries with a side of low- or nonfat ice cream, yogurt, or whipped topping (find one low in saturated fat with no hydrogenated oil).

Activity

Because you've been so good, give your body a rest. Take a nap in the afternoon or go to bed a little earlier than usual tonight. You deserve it. As you progress along in the days to come you will be slowly increasing the amount of time you work on strength training, so get into the habit now of giving your soon-to-be toned muscles a chance to rebuild. Muscles undergoing strength training need a couple of days to recuperate. When it's time to get a little stronger, you'll be well rested and ready to go again.

Mind/Body/Spirit

Many of us spend so much time worrying about deadlines at work, paying bills, shuffling kids to and from various activities, and simply trying to please others that we often neglect number one: ourselves. On that note, spend some time today pampering yourself. If you'd like, give yourself a facial at home, go get a professional manicure, or better yet indulge in a full body massage at a nearby health club. For me, nothing is more relaxing than having a trained therapist rub my tense shoulders, back, legs, and feet muscles. Try it. If money is tight, get a half-hour massage or do a you-scratch-my-back-I-scratch-yours kind of massage trade with your significant other or close friend.

FACT FUNFASTFACT FUNFASTFACT FUNFASTFACT FUNFASTFACT
UNFASTFACT FUNFASTFACT FUNFASTFACT FUNFASTFACT FUNFA

Worrying too much can actually reduce your attention span and cause lapses in your memory. Some psychologists suggest that up to ninety minutes of worry a day is normal; however, more is cause for concern. See your doctor if you think you worry too much, or simply ask yourself: "Do I solve my problems with action, or does worrying cause me to freeze in my tracks and do nothing . . . causing me to worry some more?"

Day 10 — Monday
Smoothie choice: Hawaiian Lust™

It's Monday again, so stay on course and this week is guaranteed to feel like less of a grind than ever before! To give your body the jump start it needs to power through a new and rewarding day, blend yourself together a Hawaiian Lust Smoothie. This drink is packed with calcium and plenty of the mineral manganese, which can keep your nervous system working smoothly. It is also high in vitamin C to aid in the absorption of iron and calcium. Plus, this smoothie is chock full of vitamin B_6 to help your body release more energy from the foods you eat and better utilize proteins! (See recipe on page 179.)

While you're sliding into a refreshing tropical mood, let's talk about protein. Protein is the hero that helps the body grow strong. It makes up about 20 percent of our entire weight and is an important part of our hair, nails, muscles, skin, eyes, and organs—especially our hearts and brains. Protein is a key ingredient to well-balanced nutrition, second only to water. Our immune systems also need protein so we can fight infections and to help maintain our body tissues.

Many people have been praising high protein diets for years. However, most health experts believe people are usually losing weight because they are simply eating fewer calories on these kinds of diets. There is also proof that you can eat too much protein. In fact, researchers from the University of Texas Southwestern Medical Center discovered that a high-protein, low-carbohydrate diet could increase the risk of kidney stones and bone loss. *Why does that happen?* Eating too much protein puts a strain on the kidneys—your body's water and waste management system—which may cause your kidneys to get rid of more water from the body than usual. This flush sweeps out essential minerals from the bloodstream that can cause imbalances in your body, which may lead to a heart attack.

So how much protein should you eat? For most of us, it's about 50 grams. If you're an average-built woman weighing 110 pounds, you may choose to eat about 40 grams a day. If you're 130 pounds, you could do with about 47 grams. If you're a healthy male who weighs 154 pounds, 56 grams of protein would be plenty. If you weigh 175 pounds, you need about 64 grams.

Watch your meat intake! Remember that animal products with high amounts of saturated fat have a lot of bad cholesterol (LDL) in them. In general, do not eat more than about 5 to 7 ounces of meat per day. Protein is important, but you shouldn't eat more than twice the recommended amount on any given day. One ounce of meat or fish contains about 8 grams of protein. Eight ounces of milk contains about 8 grams of protein. If you eat a 6-ounce piece of chicken for lunch (6 ounces × 8 grams of protein), that equals 48 grams of protein, which is probably pretty close to the maximum amount you need for the day.

Science tells us you should eat about 0.8 grams per kilogram of ideal body weight (1 kilogram equals 2.2 pounds), according to the U.S. Recommended Daily Allowances (RDA) for protein.

For those wanting to eat fewer or even no meat products whatsoever—for various health- and animal rights–related reasons—let's talk about a fantastic alternative protein group: nuts, beans, and legumes. Legumes are a special class of vegetables that include peas and beans. Legumes include a wide variety of delicious choices like black beans, black-eyed peas, garbanzo beans, lentils, lima beans, peanuts, green peas, and soybeans. They are an incredibly rich source of protein. Most legumes are also low in calories, low in fat, and pretty high in fiber. Plus, they may even help lower the artery-clogging bad cholesterol (LDL).

Nuts are incredible sources of protein. Walnuts also contain the essential fatty acid omega-3—which you already learned has been proven to lessen your chances of having a heart attack or cancer. In addition, "All vegetables, whole grains, and legumes provide protein, too," says Sue Havala Hobbs, R.D., author of *Vegetarian Cooking for Dummies*. So keep your nutritional options open to include those choices as well.

Nutrition

* Put a small bag of raw almonds in your glove compartment to munch on when hunger strikes. Almonds are bursting with healthy amounts of those good monounsaturated fats. Of course, because nuts are fatty they are also dense in calories, so have small, sensible handfuls at a time.
* Studies show that heart disease, cancer, and stroke—the major killers of Americans—are more likely to affect people who eat too much meat than those consuming a much more plant-based diet. Be conscious not to overdo it in the meat department today. Life is all about choices. Make yours better ones.

* Bring a bag of raw snap peas or soybean pods with you to work. They are crispy, delicious, and highly nutritious snack foods.
* Fish is a terrific source of protein. For dinner have a fresh filet of salmon, codfish, or a baked trout. For side dishes, consider having a dollop of flavorful black beans and brown rice.

Activity

Wake up earlier than usual. Go for a quick twenty-minute-or-so walk right away. Walk slowly for about five to ten minutes at first to warm up, then pick up the pace to a speed that's quicker yet still comfortable for you. On Saturday you watched a video or two featuring some strength-training exercises. After your invigorating walk, pop in your favorite video. Fast-forward to a section on leg exercises and do about ten to twenty minutes of them along with the instructor. Your legs contain the biggest muscle group in your body. When you work out your leg muscles first, those muscles will get firmer, helping you continue to burn fat even when you are resting. Commit as many of the moves as you can to memory. Exercises like squats and leg lifts can be done almost anytime and anyplace. If you have kids, invite them to join in.

Mind/Body/Spirit

Bring some outdoor splendor into your home or office with a fragrant bouquet of flowers. Having flowers around bumps up the spirit of any drab office space or cold corner in your home. Personally, I enjoy the scent of lilies, roses, and even carnations. During the course of the day stop and smell the roses, literally, every chance you get.

Day 11—Tuesday
Smoothie choice: Soy Milk Splash™

Today we're going to shine the spotlight on the amazing properties of dairy and soy. What better way to start your day than
with a mouthwatering Soy Milk Splash Smoothie. (See recipe
on page 202). Besides the creamy texture and rich taste, why
are you going to love this low-calorie eye-opener? A Soy Milk
Splash Smoothie is drenched in the mineral phosphorus to help
maintain bone density, strength, and those pearly white teeth of
yours! Plus, it's loaded with 17 grams of powerful protein, 150
percent of your RDI of vitamin C, and lots of calcium.

As you probably know, calcium is a mineral that is essential
for building healthy, strong bones and teeth. Calcium also helps
you prevent gum disease and tooth decay. Today, almost half
of all children younger than five don't get enough calcium in
their diets. And according to the National Institutes of Health,
only 13.5 percent of girls and 36.3 percent of boys in America are getting enough calcium each day, placing them at serious risk for osteoporosis and other bone diseases down the
road. Because nearly 90 percent of adult bone mass is established by the end of the teenage age range, many experts
say our nation's kids are standing center stage amidst a calcium crisis! As an adult, not enough calcium can lead to osteoporosis—a painful condition caused by the loss of bone
density. People with osteoporosis have trouble walking and
doing simple tasks. With frail, weak bones, older folks—God
rest their weary bones—are at a greater risk for hip and bone
fractures.

In addition, recent research shows that calcium directly influences whether you'll burn the food you eat as fuel or store
the food as fat. When you consume the recommended allowances for calcium (1,000 mg on average) each day—especially

in the form of food rather than supplements—your chances of slimming down quickly and easily are much greater.

What's the best way to add calcium to your diet (and your children's)? Drink an eight-ounce glass of 1 percent or nonfat milk and eat a cup of yogurt and a few slices of low-fat cheese like Swiss each day. Get calcium from other sources such as green leafy vegetables like broccoli and spinach, tofu, foods fortified with calcium, and of course by drinking soy milk and using other soy-based products.

Nutrition

* Have a cup of calcium-rich yogurt for breakfast along with a piece of fruit and a slice of whole-grain toast or bowl of cereal. Yogurt has many benefits. It acts as a cancer-fighting, antibacterial agent. It can also boost your immune system and protect you against getting future colds. Also, a daily cup of yogurt with acidophilus has been proven to prevent yeast infections in women.
* On your lunch break or on your way home from work stop at a grocery or convenience store and look for soy products. Buy ones that look appealing to you. I love lightly salted soy nuts and many soy-based ice creams!
* Tonight for dinner have some fresh steamed broccoli or asparagus spears as a side dish. And keep those liquids, especially water, coming.

Activity

If walking in the morning has been giving you the boost of energy you've been looking for, by all means keep it up. Otherwise, find about ten to twenty minutes during the day and go for a quick stroll or climb a few flights of stairs. Always warm up slowly at first. And after that you may be ready by now to pick up the pace a bit. Think brisk! For added musical motivation, put on your Walkman, find an energizing station or a CD you like, and fly like the wind!

Today is also time for a little more strength training. Free up a few moments and work on your abs for about five to fifteen minutes. Yes, those upper and lower abdominal muscles that may be hiding someone near your belt . . . that special area which can make or break an outfit. Besides helping you look a little sexier, strong ab muscles can also keep you from suffering from back pain.

To get started, lie down on the floor and wedge your feet under a solid object; a sofa will do. Place your hands behind your head, or if you haven't done a sit-up in quite some time, keep your arms along your sides. Bend your knees slightly and lift your upper body a few inches off the ground. Do a few. Rest. Repeat. Do not go all the way up to your knees as it puts too much strain on your back. Again, for extra motivation crank up some music and feel the funky beat!

Mind/Body/Spirit

Remember the last time you laughed until it hurt? You were inadvertently working out your fabulous abs! Today, pick up the phone or get together for lunch with that one person in the world who makes you laugh out loud. Tell jokes or make fun of a presidential candidate, whatever gets your funny bone jiggling. If you can't think of anyone particularly amusing, stop by the video store on your way home and rent a really funny comedy.

Day 12—Wednesday
Smoothie choice: Temple of Tangerine™

By now you know it takes more than just "an apple a day to keep the doctor away," but not that much more. All it takes is drinking plenty of refreshing water and eating more fresh fruits and vegetables, a healthy portion of protein, some nuts, beans, and legumes, and plenty of whole-grain products, which we will discuss on Friday. For now, I'll skip any kind of lecture about fruit because you already learned plenty in chapter 2, "Power Foods, Power Fruits, and Jamba Boosts!" To celebrate all the knowledge you've accumulated so far, whip yourself up a Temple of Tangerine and get happier! (See recipe on page 206.)

What else will a Temple of Tangerine do for you besides make you smile? To put it into "California surfer-speak," this totally *rad* smoothie is full of vitamin C and other *fly* antioxidants to help you fight cancer, heart disease, and avoid looking *pruned-out*.

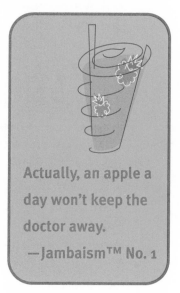

Nutrition

Actually, an apple a day won't keep the doctor away.
—Jambaism™ No. 1

✳ Keep spinning your color wheel of fruits. Remember: Each color group has a different combination of powerful antioxidants and other nutrients that will help specific yet very different parts of your mind and body. Because you started with a Temple of Tangerine have a green apple, a cup of strawberries, or a handful of white grapes as a midday snack.

✳ Try not to snack on junk food until you've at least had a piece of fruit or a handful of vegetables first. The fiber Mother Nature trapped inside her magical world of fruits and vegetables is the same fiber that makes you feel full, and it will give you more energy that lasts longer! Junk foods burn brightly and quickly, then leave you in a slump.

✳ Consider adding dried cran-raisins, plums, or apricots to a salad, rice, or meat dish at suppertime tonight.

Activity

Besides going for your usual morning or lunchtime walk (hmm, is it starting to feel like a routine?), today, it's time to spend between ten and twenty minutes doing a little strength training on your upper body. Concentrate on doing one little thing for your back, one for your shoulders, and one for your chest.

If you liked the upper-body exercises you saw on the video you rented and can remember some moves on your own, go for it. Otherwise, for your back muscles, get down on all fours and place a lightweight dumbbell or other object (a jug of laundry soap is okay) beside you at waist level. Pick up the dumbbell in one hand and support yourself with the other. Pull the weight up slowly and let it down gently for a count of about ten. Switch arms and repeat. Then do it all over again twice more.

For your shoulders, stand tall with your feet at shoulder width, grab a light dumbbell in each hand, and rest your arms at your sides. Shrug your shoulders up and down for a count of ten. Rest for a few moments. Then repeat two more times for a total count of thirty.

For your chest, lie on the floor and hold the two dumbbells next to your chest with your palms facing forward. Push the weights up slowly until you can't extend your arms any farther, repeat for a count of ten. Rest. Then repeat for a total count of thirty. That's it. That's the basis of a complete upper-body workout.

Mind/Body/Spirit

Right before you go to bed tonight sit down somewhere quiet and take a few long, deep breaths. How are you feeling? Would you feel better if you suddenly looked like a supermodel? Believe me, so would I. However, too often our feelings of self-worth are wrapped up in comparing ourselves with others. Decide right now to let those feelings go. There will always be someone better-looking and there will always be someone less attractive. There will always be someone richer and someone poorer. Someone will be smarter than you and someone will be less intelligent. Try to stop comparing yourself with others—for good. Your goals should be to increase your own sense of personal joy and to become healthier than you were yesterday.

Day 13 — Thursday
Juice choice: Vegetable Vision™

Thursday has arrived, and you're almost at the two-week mark. Wow, great job! To celebrate, start your day with a delicious, nutritious vegetable juice blend created especially for you, my Vegetable Vision—the next best thing to a Bloody Mary, if you ask me. (See recipe on page 215.) Besides the amazing ingredient lycopene—that powerful antioxidant and cancer-fighting agent tucked neatly inside every tomato on earth—this vegetable juice all-star (okay, tomatoes are actually a fruit) also has quite a spicy, nutritional spunk, compliments of the chili pepper. How can chili pepper possibly heal what ails you? Chili peppers have been shown to dissolve blood clots, break up mucus in your lungs, and open up breathing passages. Research from UCLA and other parts of the world also tell us that chili peppers can act as an expectorant and a decongestant, aid in the prevention of bronchitis, and help lessen the severity of stomach ulcers.

While we're on the topic of vegetables, here is a brief list of just some of the other best vegetables on the planet:

* **Red Bell Peppers.** All peppers are high in vitamins C and A, but red peppers are considered the *bells of the ball* because

they have more vitamin C than oranges and they contain an arsenal of cancer-fighting beta-carotenes and antioxidants.

✳ **Spinach.** Spinach is loaded with iron and folate (a B vitamin that helps fight heart disease). Spinach also contains *two* special phytochemicals (lutein and zeaxanthin) that are instrumental in keeping your eyes healthy and may even help reduce some people's chances of going blind.

✳ **Broccoli.** It's packed with beta-carotene, fiber, vitamin C, and other nutrients. Plus, according to the American Cancer Society many studies have linked eating "cruciferous" veggies like broccoli on a regular basis to a reduced risk of breast, colon, and some stomach cancers.

✳ **Sweet Potatoes.** These have more beta-carotene than any other vegetable, and they are one of the only sources of vitamin E that isn't bogged down with fat. Sweet potatoes are so good for you that the Center for Science in the Public Interest calls them "a nutritional all-star—one of the most nutritious vegetables you can eat."

✳ **Eggplants** have all sorts of phytochemicals including saponins, which studies suggest have antioxidant and anti-inflammatory properties. Eggplants can help lower bad cholesterol, too. Plus, evidence shows that eating eggplants (along with a well-balanced diet) may help halt or at least slow down the effects of aging!

Fact FunFastFact FunFastFact FunFastFact FunFastFact
unFastFact FunFastFact FunFastFact FunFastFact FunFa

Sweet potatoes are actually members of the morning glory family—as in the flower. Back in the 1500's, sweet potatoes were considered aphrodisiacs. No wonder Shakespeare was always in love!

✳ **Onions** (including chives, leeks, scallions, and shallots) are one of Mother Nature's oldest forms of medicine once used in ancient Mesopotamia to cure many sicknesses. Today we know they are bursting with many cancer-fighting agents. And shallots and yellow and red onions (not white) have been shown to thin blood, lower bad (LDL) cholesterol and raise the good (HDL), fight asthma, cure hay fever and help fight diabetes. So stop crying and eat up!

✳ **Mushrooms** (Asian and shiitake)—although not technically a vegetable but a fungus—have been revered in the Far East for centuries and used as heart medicine, longevity tonics, and as cancer remedies. Recent research by Dale Hammerschmidt, M.D., from the University of Minnesota Medical School, confirms that black mushrooms thin the blood, which may be the reason the Chinese have much lower rates of coronary heart disease. Enjoy!

More great news: Similar to fruits, each color group of the vegetable kingdom holds a unique key to better health. Be creative. Rotate your vegetables to include a red tomato for lunch, then spin into a spinach salad for dinner. Make an egg-white omelet with green bell peppers and red onions for breakfast, then steam ahead to some yellow squash and purple eggplant for dinner. Make each plate as colorful as you are!

Nutrition

✳ Keep spicing it up. Go somewhere such as a Mexican food restaurant for lunch and pour as much hot chili sauce onto your food as you can handle. In a recent British study, it was shown that spicy foods, including hot mustards and chili sauces, revved up the metabolisms of the participants by up to 25 percent! What may happen when you rev up your metabolism? That's right, you will burn more calories.

* Consider going vegetarian for the whole day (or at least partly). There are many new meat alternatives to choose from besides nuts, soy products, and green leafy vegetables as protein sources. Personally I love vegetable garden burgers and tofu stir-fry dishes.
* Keep drinking your water and rotating your rainbow of vegetable and fruit group colors every chance you get.

Activity

To break up the week, instead of going for your usual walk in the morning do something different. Today when you go to work or on an errand, give yourself extra time and park your car farther away than you have ever intentionally parked before. If you normally pick up the kids from school at three o'clock, park a few blocks away and enjoy a carefree walk with your wee ones. For an added metabolic boost yell, "Last one to the car is a rotten egg . . ." and race like wild horses. If you commute to work by subway, bus, or train get off at least one stop before you normally do. Walk briskly and enjoy the sights along the way while almost effortlessly getting in another ten- to twenty-minute aerobic workout.

In addition, do a few more sit-ups and strength-train your leg muscles for at least ten to twenty minutes or so. If you'd like, stand in place as if you were a ballet dancer and lift one leg forward for a count of ten, then to the side for ten, then toward your back for ten reps. This is an easy way to work out those spectacular leg-muscles-to-be. You can do it at work while you are on the phone or while making supper in the kitchen. And because your upper-thigh muscles are the largest muscle group in your body, when you strengthen your thighs even slightly, your newer, firmer, more toned leg muscles will also help you melt away the fat and burn off more calories faster—even at rest!

Mind/Body/Spirit

After dinner and perhaps after the kids have gone to bed, put on your PJs and pour yourself a glass of wine or open up a beer if you'd like. Then find the most inspirational piece of music you have. Maybe the *1812 Overture,* something by Elton John, or an old Aretha Franklin album rocks your world.

Turn the lights down low and light a candle. Put on the music and lie down or plop down on the most comfortable chair in the house. Shut your eyes, take a few slow deep breaths, and allow the power of the music to transport you as far away from your troubles as you can. Don't think about the past or worry about the future; simply be. Be in the moment.

Day 14 — Friday
Smoothie choice: Raspberry Rush™

Now you have made it through *two* entire weeks of eating better. You have become a little more active, perhaps even ready to razzle-dazzle the world. Wake up to a bedazzling array of nutrients and beguiling flavors inside a freshly made Raspberry Rush Smoothie, also called a Razzmatazz® at Jamba stores. (See recipe on page 200.) Besides tasting sweet and delicious, this smoothie is a dazzling source of vitamins, minerals, and antioxidants.

Today is Friday, which means we are going to concentrate on the last and largest of the five major food groups: whole grains, breads, cereals, and pastas. Most health experts ask us to eat six to eleven

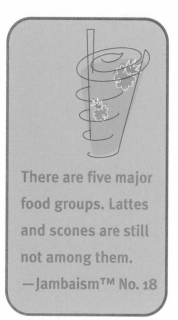

There are five major food groups. Lattes and scones are still not among them.
—Jambaism™ No. 18

> *Fact FunFastFact FunFastFact FunFastFact FunFastFact*
> *unFastFact FunFastFact FunFastFact FunFastFact FunFa*
>
> The time between when you eat something and eliminate
> it is called your ITT (intestinal transit time). Studies show
> that people whose diets are high in fiber have an ITT of
> about twelve to fourteen hours—enough time for their
> bodies to get nutrients. In the United States, where many
> people don't eat enough fiber, the average ITT is forty-
> eight to seventy-two hours, sometimes up to a full week!

servings, and there are many good reasons why. For starters, whole grains provide *complex* carbohydrates—which you may know by now are a vital source of long-lasting energy for your body and mind. Whole grains also fill us up faster, which leaves less room for less nutritious items.

Mother Nature wants us to eat lots of *whole grains* because the roughness of the fiber helps speed digestion along. In contrast, when whole grains are refined into white flours and such, the goodness of the *whole* fiber is removed and that can cause stomach problems. It may sound strange, but fiber helps you digest and eliminate foods because it is *indigestible*. In other words, just as a steel wool pad helps you scrub the grime from the bottom of a pan, your body uses fiber to scrub away toxins and push things along. If you don't have enough fiber in your tummy, food just sits there and sits there and sits there . . . if you know what I mean.

Nutrition

* Start your day with a bowl of oatmeal or high-fiber, whole-grain cereal.
* As a minimeal, feast on a few whole-wheat crackers, a cup of yogurt, and an apple.

✳   At lunchtime have a nice sandwich on dark rye or whole-wheat bread, a sliced tomato with olive oil vinaigrette, and a big glass of water.

✳   For an afternoon snack, pile up a pita with a few of your favorite vegetables and a scoop of low-fat cottage cheese.

✳   For dinner serve up a tasty serving of whole-wheat pasta primavera or spinach lasagna! Have a glass of tomato juice or red wine if you'd like.

One last nutritional note: Continue to check food labels. If a package of bread or cereal does not list whole-grain wheat, bran, or oats as the first ingredient, it probably isn't the sweetheart you want your tummy to marry.

Activity

Continue walking for twenty minutes or so in the morning or on your lunch break. Today, strengthen your triceps and biceps. Your triceps are the muscles in the back of your upper arm. Yes, the unfortunate area on certain women especially that can get a bit jiggly without proper toning. Your biceps are the area on the other side of your arm—the area bodybuilders usually flex first to show off their enormous strength. Both of these arm muscles can get toned up fairly quickly, and in doing so you will burn away the often-unsightly flab there too.

For your triceps, lean against a desk or table at waist level with one arm and pick up your light dumbbell or an object the size of a softball with the other. Lean forward slightly and raise the dumbbell behind your back until it is extended into a straight out position for a count of ten or so. Repeat with the other arm. Rest. Then do it all again for a total count of thirty.

For your biceps, stand tall with your feet at shoulder distance apart. Hold both dumbbells to your side. Curl one arm up as you've seen those bodybuilders do until the weight is almost to your chest. Allow the dumbbell to return slowly to your side.

Repeat about ten times. Switch arms and repeat. Rest. Do it all again two more times. That's it.

Mind/Body/Spirit

It's Friday and you have virtually made it two-thirds of the way toward becoming a healthier, happier, sexier you! Speaking of a sexier you, let's talk about sex appeal for a moment. In primitive times life was tough. Food was scarce and only the strongest survived. Because of those harsh conditions Mother Nature programmed us to be attracted to the healthiest-looking (read: sexy) tribesman (or -woman) we could find. Today we are all still attracted to healthy, sexy-looking mates. It's that simple.

Right now, think of three attributes that make a person sexy to you. Write them down. Now think of three things that make *you* feel sexy. Write them down. Look at your list. At some point during the day or tonight after work, do at least one thing on your list that makes you feel sexy! . . . Have fun.

Week 3—The Fun Continues

Now that your own love handles are getting closer to where *you* ideally want them to be, give yourself a big old loving hug. Congratulate your happier, more confident self on making it through two fantastic weeks of healthier living. This week, you will continue eating a wide variety of beans, nuts, and legumes. You will enjoy a colorful variety of at least five servings of fruits and vegetables every day. You will also introduce more whole-grain products, including rice and pasta, to your diet. You will strive to slow down on your consumption of foods laden with saturated fats, added sugars, and salts. And you will continue searching for more activities that are fun for *you*. Our focus this week will be on boosting your brainpower and energy levels, protecting your immune system, and, most important, reducing your stress levels.

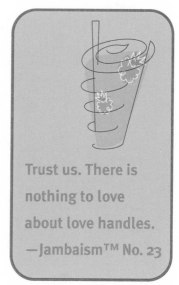

Trust us. There is nothing to love about love handles.
—Jambaism™ No. 23

Day 15—Saturday
Smoothie choice: Orange Mango Magnificence™

Let's begin the final week of your journey toward becoming a healthier, happier, sexier you with a brief discussion about stress. On the one hand, stress is simply your body's response to change. One situation that may seem stressful to you may not bother your spouse at all. For instance, I love flying in airplanes. Others get a little queasy when they are not firmly planted on the ground. My older brother gets a charge out of driving really fast, which scares the heck out of me. I like to take my time and enjoy the ride. In other words, we're all different, and we all respond to situations differently.

On the other hand, stress can set off an alarm in your brain. Your brain sends signals to many areas of your body to prepare for defensive action. Your nervous system becomes supercharged and hormones are sent to sharpen your senses, speed up your pulse, make you breathe faster, and tense up your muscles. Often this process is called your "flight or fight" response. Mother Nature programmed us that way so we could have extra energy to get out of dangerous situations. When a stressful situation keeps you in a constant state of high alert, this can put a lot of extra wear and tear on many of your biological systems, which can increase your risk of getting sick, contracting a disease, or even becoming injured.

When I first started speaking to large audiences I used to become sort of panicked, but it's not so bad anymore. Today, just thinking about speaking in front of a group of people gets me excited; it's fun. Without a little stress or excitement life would be dull.

Sure, stress can make us feel pissed off, scared, or helpless. When we are feeling stressed-out, we often have trouble sleeping. Sometimes stress can cause us to overeat, smoke, or drink too much. Other times stress can make our shoulders tense and our backs ache. The key is to learn a few ways to manage the stress in your own life, on your own terms, so that it won't lead to health problems down the road. So each day this week, in addition to a smoothie suggestion and some ideas about nutrition and staying active, I will give you a few tips on how not to let stress get your down!

The easiest and most effective way to head stress off at the pass is to keep your mind and body strong by eating a colorful array of nutritious foods and by being as active as you can. To start your day off right, why not enjoy a freshly blended Orange Mango Magnificence Smoothie. (See recipe on page 185.) Bursting with a hurricane of tangy tropical taste and ultra-high levels of antioxidants like vitamins A, C, and E, this Orange Mango Magnificence is also mighty high in vitamins B_3 and B_6, which will help your body convert the food you eat into explosive energy. It's also low in fat and it has a bounty of beta-carotene and other nutrients to keep your immune system going strong!

Nutrition

* Stress can weaken the immune system because your body perceives stress as a physical emergency. Studies show that garlic stimulates your immune functioning and helps your body generate more agents to kill tumor cells. So today eat at least one meal or an appetizer featuring garlic.
* Beta-carotene has also been shown to keep your immune system strong, so choose to eat one or more of the following today: sweet potatoes, carrots, butternut squash, or some collard greens.
* Carbohydrates like those found naturally in fruits have been shown to reduce the symptoms of stress and help calm us down. If a stressful moment comes your way, make another carbo-rich smoothie of your choice, or nibble on some other low-fat, high-carbohydrate foods such as air-popped popcorn or a couple of rice cakes, or suck on a lollipop, which does have some sugar but may keep you from eating too many other foods higher in calories.

Activity

Because this is the final Saturday on your twenty-one day journey, it's very important to keep searching for activities that you will continue to enjoy for the rest of your life. Today, I want you to look in the yellow pages or call a couple of friends and find a gym or dance studio that offers classes. Pick one and take the class. You will probably be amazed at the variety of your choices.

In most gyms you can sign up for beginning classes in:

* hip-hop, funk, reggae, and salsa aerobics
* tai chi, power yoga, and pilates
* kickboxing, karate, and tae bo
* spinning classes featuring a roomful of people on stationary bikes
* aerobics and strength-training classes specifically designed to work out your abs, thighs, buns, arms, chest, and back
* workouts that teach you how to properly use an exercise ball
* crunch cardio groove or cardio-strip aerobics
* Latin rhythm body toning
* jump rope body sculpting
* water aerobics

In many dance studios you can take classes like:

* belly-dancing, hula, and ballroom dancing
* tango, swing, and tap dancing
* New York City Ballet Workout or Ballet Boot Camp
* African healing dance and Afro-Brazilian
* country line dancing
* modern jazz

Classes can cost anywhere from absolutely *free* at some community centers and local YM/YWCAs to about ten to fifteen dollars for a dance studio class or about twenty-five dollars for a one-day pass at a gym. Beginning classes are just that—designed for beginners. You can dress comfortably, and you do not have to worry about what others will think about how you look.

Classes are fun to take. They usually last about an hour. You get to try new things and meet new people. And most important, finding activities that are enjoyable *to you* means you will stick with them.

Mind/Body/Spirit

Let's face it: As humans we are basically "pack animals." Feeling the camaraderie and spirit of being a part of a group of people is invigorating. In today's high-tech world of wizardry and long commutes into the suburbs, it's becoming easier for us to isolate ourselves, which can lead to loneliness and cause extra stress. Things that bring us together with others allow us to feel more connected, like we belong, and many health professionals such as Dr. Dean Ornish believe it is the key to emotional health. After your class today, ask someone from class or call a close friend or two and go out for a bite to eat or a smoothie.

If you've lost contact with most of your old friends—the kind you've shared the most intimate details of your life with—make a call and reconnect. He or she has probably been thinking about you and would love to get together again! When all else fails, look for a support group in your area that may interest you. Discuss anything you like but remember: The more you open up and share feelings, the happier you will have a chance to become.

Day 16—Sunday
Smoothie choice: Really . . . Raspberry™

Ah, Sunday—the pause that refreshes—and the perfect day to pop over to your nearby Jamba, if you have one, or just stay home and mix yourself a divine Really . . . Raspberry Smoothie. Why will you enjoy this winner? It's a good source of vitamin C and iron, which helps keep your blood flowing full of oxygen. It's also got fiber for healthy digestion. (See recipe on page 201.)

Nutrition

* Because you've been so good, indulge one of your food fantasies for breakfast. Bake a plate of cinnamon buns or go out for eggs Benedict. It's important to eat right most of the time but life isn't as much fun if you don't let loose every once in a while! Plus, even nuns have bad habits!

* Keep drinking plenty of water throughout the day. Consider having a glass of refreshing iced tea with a lemon wedge and a sprig of fresh mint *early* in the day—caffeine can linger in your system for up to ten hours, and you need your sleep.

* For dinner, go Mediterranean. Many leading health experts have hailed the Mediterranean diet because it is abundant in seafood, olive oil, multicolored fruits and vegetables, and even red wine. Doesn't cranberry-ginger salmon, chicken pie with apricots, and gazpacho with roasted cherry tomatoes sound enticing? One instantaneous way to get hundreds of recipes *for free* is to go on line and type in a key word or two such as: "Mediterranean recipes." Try it right now and see for yourself!

Activity

If you have stayed on course for the last two weeks, you may want to rest for most of the day. However, if you've missed a couple of ten-minute aerobic sessions here or a brief strength-training session there, call a few friends and get together at a nearby park. If you have kids, bring them along and invite some of their friends as well. Be active. Enjoy a game of softball, kickball, tag, touch football, or volleyball. Playing outdoor sports with friends is a blast. It allows you to be active for hours without feeling like it's a burden. If you don't want to do anything strenuous, go for a leisurely stroll.

Mind/Body/Spirit

To ensure that you have a more relaxing, less stressed-out week: Later in the day, make a list of all the things you have to do this week. Take a good, long look at your list. Are there any things that really aren't that important? Is there something on your list that someone else might actually be happy to do? Is there anything on your list that you could afford to pay someone to do? Could you trade services with a neighbor, perhaps alternating who takes the kids to school?

Cross one, two, or as many things off your list as you feel comfortable with. For the rest of today and throughout the week stop promising to do too much. Give yourself more time to do the things you want to do, such as getting more physically fit and sleeping eight hours every night. Allow yourself more time to pack healthier lunches and things to snack on for yourself and your children. Keep remembering: Five smaller meals a day can help you stay energized and control your weight. Practice saying "No," or "I'll think about it. Let me get back to you on that."

Day 17 — Monday
Smoothie choice: I've Gone Totally Guava™

You're in the home stretch now! It's Monday of the final week. You're probably looking and feeling better than you have for a long time. To help you power through another fun-filled and less-stressed-out day, start off by fortifying your body with some key nutrients found neatly tucked inside a I've Gone Totally Guava Smoothie! (See recipe on page 181.)

Nutrition

* One item often overlooked as a culprit when it comes to increasing your stress levels is caffeine. Sure, a couple of cups of coffee (or between 250 and 300 mg of caffeine) are generally not a problem. In fact, caffeine can give us a kick, improve our mood, and help us work out harder. However, too much of a good thing can cause nervousness, restlessness, and anxiety. So watch out because one extra-large coffee from many popular coffeehouses may contain up to 500 mg of nerve-rattling caffeine! Also, certain fancy frozen coffee drinks can contain up to 700 calories, 100 from the whipped cream alone! So today, drink a little less coffee than usual or switch to a delightful, cancer-fighting cup of green or black tea, which has a lot less caffeine (about 35 to 50 mg).
* Fruits and vegetables rich in beta-carotene can boost your body's natural defense system against such attackers as bacterial and viral infections, so bring a bag of already-prepared carrots with you wherever you go.
* To further help keep your immune system strong, concentrate on taking it easy on foods with too many saturated fats like red meat or "whole" dairy products. In a recent study at the University of Massachusetts Medical School it was found that decreasing the bad fats in your diet can boost the "natural killer cell activity" that snuffs out free radicals before they can do damage.

Activity

Go for your usual walk in the morning or during your lunch break. Try to increase your time to about fifteen minutes to half an hour and consider walking slightly faster than last week. Don't go overboard. Warm up by walking slowly at first. Even after you pick up the pace you should be able to chat on your cell phone or talk with a friend while walking. If you are out of breath, you are working too hard.

In addition, try to squeeze in three ten-minute sessions of leg exercises. Do a few squats, lunges, and leg lifts while you are talking on the phone or preparing a meal. Squats are basically exactly what they sound like: Stand up with your feet at shoulder distance apart, keep your back straight, and squat down as low as you can comfortably go. Hold on to an object for balance if you like. Lunges are what they sound like, too: Stand up and put one leg ahead of you by about two feet. Lunge forward. Leg lifts are those ballet-type moves you did last Thursday. Pop on your headphones for added motivation whenever you need it.

Mind/Body/Spirit

Have you ever watched the eleven o'clock news and gotten so wound up that you had trouble falling asleep? Have you ever skimmed the pages of a beauty magazine only to find yourself feeling awful because the women were so thin and gorgeous you felt like crap? There's no doubt about it; watching the news and thumbing through beauty magazines can cause us to get very stressed. Today, consider taking break from both and just see how much better you feel.

Obviously if something serious is going on in the world, go ahead and check in to see what's up. But if you can help it, do not let the negativity of the world's news or how beautiful anyone else looks get you down. A little progress toward becoming healthier, happier, and sexier is better than doing nothing.

Day 18—Tuesday
Smoothie choice: Cranberry Bogs Forever™

Today, if you want to stay smart, maintain your vision, and learn another way to help recapture the smooth skin of your youth, treat your taste buds and body to a Cranberry Bogs Forever Smoothie. What else is behind its hidden powers? This smoothie is crammed with high levels of calcium and vitamin C, and it's a good source of vitamin B_2, a.k.a. riboflavin. Riboflavin is an important vitamin because it helps you process energy from food. It also strengthens your blood and is essential for healthy eyes. This Cranberry Bogs Forever Smoothie is also filled with vitamin B_6 that can help protect you against future infections! (See recipe on page 172.)

Nutrition

* Speaking of infections, blueberries can also help block infectious bacteria. So have a handful of fresh (or recently thawed) blueberries with a cup of yogurt or on top of a bowl of whole-wheat cereal in the morning.
* Bladder infections affect many more women than men. To help you combat future bladder infections, drink another small glass of cranberry juice later in the day or add dried cranberries to a wild-rice side dish or salad for dinner tonight.
* Fluids can keep your system clean, so keep drinking water and eating plenty of water-rich fruits and vegetables.

Activity

Today's activity is called interval training, and I like it because it can turn a same-old, same-old walk into something a whole lot more exciting. Here's how it works: Start walking for five 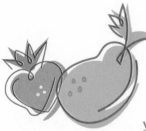 minutes at a relaxing pace to warm up your muscles. Then increase your speed until you are almost jogging. Continue for three to five minutes and then slow back down to a more easygoing pace for five to ten minutes, or whatever feels right for you. After you catch your breath, do it all over again for twenty to forty minutes. Alternating like this—from slow to fast and back—is extra fun because it breaks things up, which means you can work out for longer periods of time without feeling like it's a chore. This kind of workout also helps you burn more calories and increase your aerobic "with oxygen" capacity.

Mind/Body/Spirit

Instead of doing something for yourself or showing just one person that you care, go global! Today spend time thinking about one small thing you could do that would contribute to the betterment of the planet. Just as your body is the only one you've got, the earth is the only inhabitable planet we've got! Consider getting involved in a global charity soon as a volunteer or donating a couple of bucks. A few examples of charities I admire are: UNICEF—a charity dedicated to saving children's lives and helping build better futures through health, nutrition, clean water, education, and emergency relief fund; Greenpeace—a nonprofit dedicated to helping our global environment; and Habitat for Humanity—a charity group that works to build shelter for families and communities in need.

Day 19 — Wednesday
Smoothie choice: Be Boysenberried™

Only two more days to go! Congratulations! To help celebrate your achievement, make a Be Boysenberried Smoothie first thing in the morning or the moment you get home from work. (See recipe on page 167.) Why will you enjoy this smoothie? The flavorful berries are full of vitamin C, which is essential for helping your body to heal. This smoothie champion is also packed with 38 percent of your daily fiber. And the bananas contain plenty of vitamin B_6 to help keep your nervous system and brain functioning at their very best.

Nutrition

∗ Speaking of brainpower, another way you can maximize your alertness is to eat protein first thing in the morning. So scramble up a couple of egg whites, eat a cup of yogurt, or enjoy a couple of slices of low-fat lunch meat.

∗ For a midmorning brain-boosting mini-meal try a slice of cantaloupe along with a handful of pecans, peanuts, or almonds.

∗ The good (omega-3) fats found in fish are used by your brain to nourish the cells involved in thought and emotion, so have a tuna sandwich on rye or a broiled filet of salmon for lunch. If you normally mix tuna with lots of mayo, beware: Saturated fat is a brain downer, so go light or try eating your tuna with lemon juice, chopped carrots, pickles, and diced red onions.

∗ For a mid-afternoon mental pick-me-up have a cup of protein-rich low-fat cottage cheese with sliced tomatoes and a glass of iced tea on the side.

∗ Keep drinking your *agua* (water), señor or señorita.

Activity

To keep your brain from getting foggy, you need to keep pumping blood into it. Free up a few moments to exercise your brain muscles with a crossword puzzle, or play a board game with your kids after dinner. Continue walking for about fifteen to thirty minutes. At some point do about fifteen to thirty minutes of strength-training isometric exercises—the kind that use your body as resistance. Remember the old phrase "We must, we must, we must increase our bust"? That is an isometric exercise in which you clasp your hands in front of your chest and push them together and then pull them apart. Another example would be to stand and face a wall. Press your fist into the wall,

FACT FUNFASTFACT FUNFASTFACT FUNFASTFACT FUNFASTFACT
UNFASTFACT FUNFASTFACT FUNFASTFACT FUNFASTFACT FUNFA

Want to maximize your mind's potential? Your brain needs more oxygen than any other organ, so it's extra sensitive to oxidation (the process that turns an apple brown after cutting into it). To neutralize the damage eat more foods rich in antioxidants such as beets, grape juice, berries, red peppers, spinach, prunes, citrus fruits, and carrots!

hold for a few seconds, and repeat for a count of ten. Get creative. Have fun. You can do an isometric exercise almost anywhere, including standing in line, talking on the phone, or drying off with a towel after a shower.

Mind/Body/Spirit

No doubt about it: Outside forces can be very mentally upsetting—especially things like a boss yelling at you, or getting a flat tire on the way to work when you're already ten minutes late! Today, whenever a stressful situation presents itself, keep reminding yourself that it's not the outside force that is important; it's how you react to it. Keep trying to accept those things you cannot change. If something major happens, try not to burden yourself with the entire weight of the problem. Call a friend or family member and talk it out.

Day 20—Thursday
Smoothie choice: Orange and Papaya Partnership™

Only one more day to go. Can you believe it? To squeeze the most out of your day, begin by mixing yourself a sensational Orange and Papaya Partnership Smoothie. Not only is this liquid powerhouse packed with the natural goodness of orange juice, pears, and papayas for long-lasting energy; it also contains plenty of the mineral manganese. Manganese has many functions. It helps you metabolize proteins, fats, and carbs. It helps promote a healthy nervous system and can help people with blood sugar problems. Manganese is also vital to a strong immune system, and it can help you lessen the signs of aging! (See recipe on page 182.)

Nutrition

* Whole grains such as oatmeal, buckwheat, and whole wheat are terrific sources of manganese too. Have a couple of buckwheat pancakes for breakfast or a quick bowl of whole-wheat cereal.
* For a mini midmorning meal enjoy a cup of yogurt, a slice of honeydew melon, and a small handful of hazelnuts or pecans that are also rich sources of antiaging manganese.
* For lunch add a couple of slices of avocado to whatever floats your boat and remember the number-one key to younger-looking skin is oxygen and hydration; so keep drinking your water to hydrate and keep oxygenating your system through exercise.
* Continue eating five small meals each day and five to nine servings of fruits and veggies.

Activity

Researchers now know that people who exercise regularly slow down their aging process. To continue on your path toward looking and feeling younger than ever, remember to stay active. Keep things interesting today by breaking up your workout session into two fifteen- to thirty-minute workouts or three ten- to twenty-minute periods. And practice interval training as you go as you did on Tuesday—only this time walk for a few minutes at a somewhat leisurely pace, then burst into a few calisthenics or isometric exercise, such as jumping jacks, push-ups (wall push-ups or knee push-ups are fine), and step-ups. Step-ups simply involve stepping up on a curb, sturdy bench, or stair on one foot, then the other, for a count of ten for each. To help motivate you, put on your headphones and switch from a slow song to a fast one and then back again. You will be amazed at how much fun this is as well as how much energy you have long afterward!

Mind/Body/Spirit

Being stressed-out can take a toll on us emotionally, mentally, and spiritually. It can also make us age a whole lot quicker. Because we're all unique, different triggers set us off; certain things lead us toward becoming angry, upset, or stressed-out. This morning while you are bathing and grooming think of things in your own life that really get your goat. Maybe rush-hour traffic drives you nuts or you have too much work.

After you have thought of a few things that drive you batty, think of a few solutions so that in the near future those things won't bother you because you have successfully avoided them! If horrible traffic in the morning stresses you out, join a gym near work and leave before traffic gets bad. When work gets overwhelming, don't overwork. Take breaks and you'll be more productive.

Day 21—Friday
Smoothie choice: Holistic Honeydew™

Congratulations! You have finally arrived. Obviously, this calls for a celebration, so this morning blend yourself a cool, refreshing Holistic Honeydew Smoothie. (See recipe on page 180.) You deserve it! While you're savoring this nutritional firecracker, reflect on all that you have learned about fresh fruits, vegetables, legumes, nuts, proteins, and dairy products. Think about how much you now know about different kinds of exercises and how vital staying active is to your health, happiness, and sex appeal.

Nutrition

* Because the final day of this twenty-one-day journey is actually the beginning of a lifetime of healthier, more vibrant living, feel free to eat and drink as you feel is right for you.
* You'll probably want each of your five smaller meals to be bursting with brightly colored fresh fruits and flavorful vegetables.
* You'll probably choose whole-grain products over highly refined ones.
* You'll probably yearn for protein choices with less saturated fat and more essential fatty acids like those found in fish.
* You'll probably want to have a few beans, snap peas, or another legume at more meals.
* And you'll probably not feel right unless you drink enough you-know-what (yes, *water*).

Activity

It's the final day of the program. If you started walking on day one and have continued faithfully on course, walking has become routine, a new habit, the way you suddenly define yourself. Doesn't it feel good to say "Oh, I walk every day to stay fit" or "No thanks, I don't have time to watch *Survivor Twenty-Three*, I'm going for my invigorating sunset walk in the park"?

Because you have been so good, your activity for the day is "your choice." That's right, at this point you've learned all sorts of new ways to become more active . . . walking, dancing, weight lifting, interval training, and more. Now and every day forward it's time for you to decide for yourself which activities you want to do! My only suggestions at this point are for you to keep striving to exercise anywhere from twenty minutes to a full hour, five or six days a week. Keep changing your routine. Mix things up. Take more classes. Learn a new sport. Join a team. Keep a basketball and a tennis racket in the trunk of your car. Keep busy. Keep surprising your mind, body, and spirit. You know the rewards are well worth your time!

Mind/Body/Spirit

In case you forgot, Jamba is derived from a West African word that translates as "Celebrate!" And because many studies, including a recent one from Tel Aviv University in Israel, show that having a glass of wine (especially red wine, because of the powerful antioxidants), beer, or a mixed drink or two can thin your blood and keep your heart healthy, drink up! Of course, I am *not* suggesting you become a hard drinker; I am just saying that you have been a very good girl or boy and you deserve to celebrate. A healthy lifestyle *can* include the moderate consumption of alcohol or no consumption whatsoever. It's your choice. But whatever you decide, have a party! Invite a few friends over to discuss your success. Dance in your living room, or in the backyard. Be with people you enjoy. Feel good about what you have accomplished. Have confidence that your life is now on a happier, healthier, sexier course—for good!

What Now?

At the end of the day, the future of your health is in *your* hands. You can choose to pork out on junk foods 24/7 and never work out. But by now you know what will probably happen to your

precious mind, body, and spirit if you spiral down that dangerous fork in the road.

Or, you can choose to embrace your inner Jamba by running,
skipping, and jumping for joy. You can hike, bike, or dance
around the living room in your undies if you want. You can continue choosing to eat a kaleidoscope of colorful foods and delicious beverages. You can reap amazing
rewards by enjoying a wide assortment of
fresh fruits and vegetables, a select portion of leaner cuts of meat, and tender
slices of savory fish. You can enjoy small
handfuls of almonds, sunflower seeds,
and other nuts, and a tantalizing array
of lentils, beans, legumes, and succulent
sweet peas. You can boost your metabolism, strengthen your heart, and prevent
all sorts of diseases just by choosing to eat
more luscious legumes, fewer items laden
with saturated fats, little to no hydrogenated or partially hydrogenated oils,
and ample portions of whole-grain prod-
ucts. You can feel more energized, and better about yourself,
within a few weeks and months of beginning an exercise program that is fun for you.

> Two hundred and fifty thousand American deaths are due to a lack of regular physical activity.
>
> —American Heart Association, 2002

Still not sure how, why, or where? David Flemming, the Centers for Disease Control deputy director for science and public
health urges, "People of all ages can benefit from being more
active. There are many small things that people can do to increase their physical activity. People can take the stairs instead
of the elevator or even park the car farther away at the grocery
store." Tommy G. Thompson, the secretary of Health and Human Services, says, "You don't have to work up a big sweat at
the gym or become a long-distance runner. Just thirty minutes
of walking a day, five days a week, can significantly improve

your health. Playing with your kids in the backyard for an hour each day can help the whole family stay healthy." Even President Bush suggests, "Just a stroll in the park for a reasonable period of time is exercise, and it's good for you."

Want even more easy ideas on how to add movement to your life?

Home, Sweet, Active Home

✻ While chatting on your cell phone, choose to walk around the block or even around the inside of your house. If you're talking on a landline do a few sit-ups or squats or stand up during your conversations. Anything *active* you do burns more calories than *nothing.*

✻ Let your green thumb blossom. Plant a garden, pick some flowers (no, not the neighbors'!), pull a few weeds, or mow the friggin' lawn. FYI: Riding a mower doesn't count, cowboy!

✻ If you don't already have a dog, consider adopting one from a shelter. That way, you might be more apt to take Rover (and yourself) for a stroll every day. Plus, studies show a pet can help you feel less stressed-out.

✻ Leave your car in park more often. Walk, skip, or ride your bike to the mall or corner store instead of driving whenever you possibly can.

✻ Buy a treadmill or stationary bike and pedal your way to better fitness while reading or watching your favorite TV shows.

✻ If you can't seem to exercise during your workweek, make up for a little lost time on the weekends by playing volleyball, golfing, or going somewhere to sightsee on foot.

Be More Active at Work

✳ As often as possible, take short breaks and stroll into the great outdoors with coworkers for brief meetings or to brainstorm ideas together. Studies show that if you take a ten- to fifteen-minute break every few hours you can increase your brainpower by almost 25 percent!

✳ Walk down the hall to speak with people instead of just picking up the phone or e-mailing.

✳ While on business trips, book yourself into hotels with pools, gyms, and spas. Get in a few nice long workouts while away.

✳ If you haven't already done so, join a gym near work. Take yoga, step, or aerobics classes in the morning before work. For the more adventurous minded, try a Saturday-afternoon cardio striptease class. Or simply pump some iron and jog for half an hour after work. If you are a quick-change artist, pop in for a mini lunchtime sweat session and shower.

✳ In between appointments or phone calls get down and do a few push-ups, sit-ups, or squats. No one has to know what goes on behind your closed door, eh?

Play Time in Your Free Time

✳ If you enjoy watching sports, take it to the next level. In fact, take a baseball, two gloves, and a bat over to your friend's house to watch a game. At halftime run out into the yard and Jamba!

✳ Plan your vacations so you can do active things like skiing, hiking, mountain climbing, parasailing, biking, or just strolling though a beautiful city like Paris, New York, San Francisco, Vancouver, or Chicago.

✳ Take up a new sport. Ever tried tennis, scuba diving, or martial arts?

Remember, the fate of your mind, body, and spirit is in *your* hands. Choose wisely, Little Weed-Hopper. Decide to become more active and get to it. Again, you don't have to become a basketball superstar. You don't have to run marathons. You don't have to swim the English Channel—twice! You simply need to add a little more movement to your life. Five minutes here, twenty minutes there—combined with a colorful variety of more nutritious food and smooth beverage choices—may just add up to your own personally and perfectly blended recipe for a healthier, happier, sexier you.

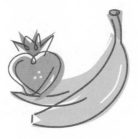

Chapter 5

Delicious Smoothie Recipes

Blending a smoothie can be a true art form. Listen and watch your smoothie as it blends. Here is a checklist for blending the perfect smoothie.

1. Pour in measured amount of liquid (juice, soy milk, etc.).
2. Add frozen ingredients such as hard-packed yogurt, sherbet, etc., except ice.
3. Add fresh or frozen fruit.
4. Add a boost such as powdered soy protein.
5. Add ice.
6. Double check the smoothie to make sure that you have all the right ingredients.
7. Begin blending on low. Listen and watch what happens.
8. After about 30 seconds blend on high until you "see the whirl in the center of the blender cup."
9. Take lid off and tap on the side of the blender cup while pouring.

10. For the proper thickness, your smoothie should form a mound in the cup. This is the Jamba standard for most smoothies.

Tips

1. Too thick? Add more liquid.
2. Too thin? Add more frozen ingredients.
3. Chunky, weird matter? Reblend and recheck for proper ingredients!
4. The blades stop to catch the ingredients? Take blender cup off and give it one good shake. Restart the blender. Repeat if necessary.
5. *Big warning:* Always turn the blender off before putting anything in it. Especially your hands, Houdini!

Ah . . . Apples and Peaches™

1 cup apple juice

½ cup pears

1 cup peaches

1 cup orange sherbet

½ cup ice

. . . .

Nutritional Information

Calories 510   Calories from fat 40

Total fat 4.5g   7%

Saturated fat 2.5 g   7%

Cholesterol 10 mg   4%

Sodium 105 mg   4%

Total carbohydrates 121 g   40%

Dietary fiber 5 g   22%

Sugars 101 g

Protein 4 g

Vitamin A 20%

Vitamin C 35%

Calcium 15%

Iron 4%

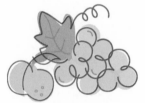

Aloha Pineapple™

¾ cup pineapple juice

¼ cup plain yogurt

½ cup bananas

1 cup strawberries

1 cup pineapple sherbet

½ cup ice

. . . .

Nutritional Information

Calories 490   Calories from fat 35

Total fat 3.5 g   6%

Saturated fat 2 g   9%

Cholesterol 10 mg   4%

Sodium 95 mg   4%

Total carbohydrates 107 g   36%

Dietary fiber 3 g   12%

Sugars 88 g

Protein 7 g

Vitamin A 10%

Vitamin C 230%

Calcium 20%

Iron 4%

Apple Affair™

1 cup apple juice

1 cup bananas

½ cup raspberries

1 cup raspberry sherbet

½ cup ice

. . . .

Nutritional Information

Calories 510   Calories from fat 10

Total fat 1 g   2%

Saturated fat 0 g   0%

Cholesterol 0 mg   0%

Sodium 55 mg   2%

Total carbohydrates 122 g   41%

Dietary fiber 8 g   33%

Sugars 109 g

Protein 4 g

Vitamin A 6%

Vitamin C 50%

Calcium 10%

Iron 4%

Apple Attraction™

1 cup apple juice

½ cup pears

1 cup nectarines

1 cup orange sherbet

½ cup ice

. . . .

Nutritional Information

Calories 500   Calories from fat 45

Total fat 5 g   8%

Saturated fat 2.5 g   12%

Cholesterol 10 mg   4%

Sodium 105 mg   4%

Total carbohydrates 118   39%

Dietary fiber 4 g   17%

Sugars 100 g

Protein 4 g

Vitamin A 25%

Vitamin C 30%

Calcium 15%

Iron 4%

Apple Kiwi Kosmo™

1 cup apple juice

½ cup pears

1 cup kiwis

1 cup lime sherbet

½ cup ice

. . . .

Nutritional Information

Calories 480   Calories from fat 25

Total fat 3 g   5%

Saturated fat 1.5 g   7%

Cholesterol 10 mg   3%

Sodium 20 mg   0%

Total carbohydrates 114 g   38%

Dietary fiber 7 g   30%

Sugars 104 g

Protein 4g

Vitamin A 6%

Vitamin C 190%

Calcium 15%

Iron 4%

Apple Plum Player™

1 cup apple juice

½ cup pears

1 cup plums

1 cup raspberry sherbet

½ cup ice

. . . .

Nutritional Information

Calories 480   Calories from fat 10

Total fat 1.5 g   2%

Saturated fat 0 g   0%

Cholesterol 0 mg   0%

Sodium 50 mg   2%

Total carbohydrates 114 g   38%

Dietary fiber 5 g   19%

Sugars 104 g

Protein 5 g

Vitamin A 10%

Vitamin C 35%

Calcium 10%

Iron 2%

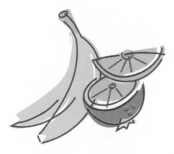

Apricot Affinity™

1 cup apple juice

½ cup pears

1 cup apricots

1 cup nonfat vanilla frozen yogurt

½ cup ice

. . . .

Nutritional Information

Calories 420   Calories from fat 10

Total fat 1 g   2%

Saturated fat 0 g   0%

Cholesterol 5 mg   0%

Sodium 140 mg   6%

Total carbohydrates 95 g   32%

Dietary fiber 6 g   23%

Sugars 89 g

Protein 13 g

Vitamin A 100%

Vitamin C 40%

Calcium 35%

Iron 6%

Be Boysenberried™

1 cup apple juice

½ cup bananas

1 cup boysenberries

1 cup nonfat vanilla frozen yogurt

½ cup ice

. . . .

Nutritional Information

Calories 440   Calories from fat 10

Total fat 1 g   2%

Saturated fat 0 g   0%

Cholesterol 5 mg   1%

Sodium 140 mg   6%

Total carbohydrates 103 g   34%

Dietary fiber 9 g   38%

Sugars 92 g

Protein 11 g

Vitamin A 6%

Vitamin C 60%

Calcium 40%

Iron 6%

Boysenberry Blitz™

1 cup boysenberry cider

½ cup boysenberries

½ cup blueberries

½ cup bananas

1 cup nonfat vanilla frozen yogurt

½ cup ice

. . . .

Nutritional Information

Calories 490   Calories from fat 1.5

Total fat 1.5 g   2%

Saturated fat 0 g   0%

Cholesterol 5 mg   1%

Sodium 140 mg   6%

Total carbohydrates 112 g   37%

Dietary fiber 9 g   35%

Sugars 97 g

Protein 14 g

Vitamin A 4%

Vitamin C 25%

Calcium 40%

Iron 10%

Cantaloupe Caress™

1 cup pear juice

½ cup bananas

1 cup cantaloupe

1 cup orange sherbet

½ cup ice

. . . .

Nutritional Information

Calories 520   Calories from fat 45

Total fat 4.5 g   7%

Saturated fat 2.5 g   12%

Cholesterol 10 mg   4%

Sodium 140 mg   6%

Total carbohydrates 124 g   41%

Dietary fiber 4 g   17%

Sugars 99 g

Protein 5 g

Vitamin A 130%

Vitamin C 270%

Calcium 15%

Iron 8%

Cherish the Cherries™

1 cup cherry cider

1 cup cherries

½ cup bananas

1 cup nonfat vanilla frozen yogurt

½ cup ice

. . . .

Nutritional Information

Calories 550   Calories from fat 5

Total fat 0.5 g   1%

Saturated fat 0 g   0%

Cholesterol 5 mg   1%

Sodium 160 mg   7%

Total carbohydrates 129 g   43%

Dietary fiber 3 g   12%

Sugars 122 g

Protein 13 g

Vitamin A 8%

Vitamin C 120%

Calcium 35%

Iron 8%

Cherry Chicle™

1 cup cherry cider

1 cup pears

½ cup strawberries

1 cup raspberry sherbet

½ cup ice

. . . .

Nutritional Information

Calories 500   Calories from fat 30

Total fat 3 g   5%

Saturated fat 1 g   6%

Cholesterol 10 mg   3%

Sodium 80 mg   3%

Total carbohydrates 120 g   40%

Dietary fiber 5g   22%

Sugars 106 g

Protein 3 g

Vitamin A 2%

Vitamin C 140%

Calcium 10%

Iron 10%

Cranberry Bogs Forever™

¾ cup cranberry juice

¼ cup plain yogurt

1 cup strawberries

½ cup blueberries

1 cup raspberry sherbet

½ cup ice

. . . .

Nutritional Information

Calories 470   Calories from fat 15

Total fat 2 g   3%

Saturated fat 0.5 g   3%

Cholesterol 5 mg   1%

Sodium 100 mg   4%

Total carbohydrates 104 g   35%

Dietary fiber 2 g   8%

Sugars 79 g

Protein 7 g

Vitamin A 4%

Vitamin C 230%

Calcium 20%

Iron 6%

Date Dazzle™

1 cup soy milk

1 cup bananas

½ cup dates

1 cup nonfat vanilla frozen yogurt

½ cup ice

. . . .

Nutritional Information

Calories 650   Calories from fat 50

Total fat 6 g   9%

Saturated fat 1 g   6%

Cholesterol 5 mg   1%

Sodium 170 mg   7%

Total carbohydrates 143 g   48%

Dietary fiber 11 g   46%

Sugars 123 g

Protein 20 g

Vitamin A 6%

Vitamin C 25%

Calcium 40%

Iron 15%

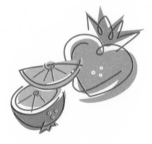

Giddy Guava™

1 cup guava nectar

½ cup bananas

1 cup mangos

1 cup nonfat vanilla frozen yogurt

½ cup ice

. . . .

Nutritional Information

Calories 520   Calories from fat 10

Total fat 1.5 g   2%

Saturated fat 0.5 g   3%

Cholesterol 5 mg   1%

Sodium 140 mg   6%

Total carbohydrates 122 g   41%

Dietary fiber 7 g   27%

Sugars 112 g

Protein 12 g

Vitamin A 130%

Vitamin C 170%

Calcium 35%

Iron 4%

Goodness Grape-cious™

1 cup grape juice

1 cup strawberries

½ cup plums

1 cup raspberry sherbet

½ cup ice

. . . .

Nutritional Information

Calories 480   Calories from fat 10

Total fat 1 g   2%

Saturated fat 0 g   0%

Cholesterol 0 mg   0%

Sodium 50 mg   2%

Total carbohydrates 109 g   36%

Dietary fiber 3 g   10%

Sugars 58 g

Protein 5 g

Vitamin A 8%

Vitamin C 150%

Calcium 15%

Iron 6%

Grape Cherry Catapult™

1 cup grape juice

½ cup pears

1 cup cherries

1 cup nonfat vanilla frozen yogurt

½ cup ice

. . . .

Nutritional Information

Calories 500   Calories from fat 20

Total fat 2 g   3%

Saturated fat 0.5 g   3%

Cholesterol 5 mg   1%

Sodium 140 mg   6%

Total carbohydrates 112 g   37%

Dietary fiber 6 g   22%

Sugars 67 g

Protein 13 g

Vitamin A 8%

Vitamin C 25%

Calcium 40%

Iron 8%

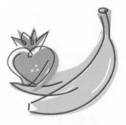

Grapefruit Grove™

1 cup grapefruit juice

1 cup pears

½ cup honeydew melon

1 cup lime sherbet

½ cup ice

. . . .

Nutritional Information

Calories 480   Calories from fat 25

Total fat 3 g   4%

Saturated fat 1.5 g   7%

Cholesterol 10 mg   3%

Sodium 10 mg   1%

Total carbohydrates 113 g   38%

Dietary fiber 5 g   19%

Sugars 103 g

Protein 3 g

Vitamin A 2%

Vitamin C 50%

Calcium 10%

Iron 2%

Growin' Grapefruits™

1 cup grapefruit juice

1 cup pears

½ cup kiwis

1 cup raspberry sherbet

½ cup ice

. . . .

Nutritional Information

Calories 500   Calories from fat 10

Total fat 1 g   2%

Saturated fat 0 g   0%

Cholesterol 0 mg   0%

Sodium 45 mg   2%

Total carbohydrates 116 g   39%

Dietary fiber 7 g   27%

Sugars 103 g

Protein 3 g

Vitamin A 4%

Vitamin C 110%

Calcium 10%

Iron 4%

Hawaiian Lust™

1 cup pineapple juice

1 cup strawberries

½ cup bananas

2 tablespoons coconut

1 cup nonfat vanilla frozen yogurt

½ cup ice

. . . .

Nutritional Information

Calories 490   Calories from fat 45

Total fat 5 g   8%

Saturated fat 4.5 g   22%

Cholesterol 5 mg   1%

Sodium 180 mg   7%

Total carbohydrates 102 g   34%

Dietary fiber 4 g   14%

Sugars 81 g

Protein 11 g

Vitamin A 10%

Vitamin C 250%

Calcium 35%

Iron 6%

Holistic Honeydew™

1 cup pear juice

1 cup kiwis

½ cup honeydew melon

1 cup nonfat vanilla frozen yogurt

½ cup ice

. . . .

Nutritional Information

Calories 440   Calories from fat 10

Total fat 1.5 g   2%

Saturated fat 0 g   0%

Cholesterol 5 mg   1%

Sodium 160 mg   7%

Total carbohydrates 100 g   33%

Dietary fiber 6 g   25%

Sugars 86 g

Protein 12 g

Vitamin A 6%

Vitamin C 370%

Calcium 40%

Iron 8%

I've Gone Totally Guava™

1 cup guava nectar

1 cup bananas

½ cup peaches

1 cup pineapple sherbet

½ cup ice

. . . .

Nutritional Information

Calories 560   Calories from fat 25

Total fat 3 g   4%

Saturated fat 1.5 g   7%

Cholesterol 5 mg   2%

Sodium 50 mg   2%

Total carbohydrates 135 g   45%

Dietary fiber 8 g   30%

Sugars 123 g

Protein 5 g

Vitamin A 15%

Vitamin C 110%

Calcium 10%

Iron 4%

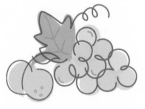

Orange and Papaya Partnership™

1 cup orange juice

½ cup pears

1 cup papayas

1 cup pineapple sherbet

½ cup ice

. . . .

Nutritional Information

Calories 450   Calories from fat 25

Total fat 3 g   4%

Saturated fat 1.5 g   6%

Cholesterol 5 mg   2%

Sodium 50 mg   2%

Total carbohydrates 104 g   35%

Dietary fiber 5 g   21%

Sugars 94 g

Protein 5 g

Vitamin A 20%

Vitamin C 360%

Calcium 15%

Iron 4%

Orange Apricot Appetite™

1 cup orange juice

½ cup bananas

1 cup apricots

1 cup nonfat vanilla frozen yogurt

½ cup ice

. . . .

Nutritional Information

Calories 400   Calories from fat 15

Total fat 1.5 g   3%

Saturated fat 0 g   0%

Cholesterol 5 mg   1%

Sodium 135 mg   6%

Total carbohydrates 87 g   29%

Dietary fiber 5 g   19%

Sugars 78 g

Protein 14 g

Vitamin A 100%

Vitamin C 300%

Calcium 40%

Iron 10%

Orange Kiwi . . . Okay™

1 cup orange juice

1 cup strawberries

½ cup kiwis

1 cup raspberry sherbet

½ cup ice

. . . .

Nutritional Information

Calories 430   Calories from fat 10

Total fat 1.5 g   2%

Saturated fat 0 g   0%

Cholesterol 0 mg   0%

Sodium 50 mg   2%

Total carbohydrates 98 g   33%

Dietary fiber 4 g   17%

Sugars 83 g

Protein 5 g

Vitamin A 15%

Vitamin C 440%

Calcium 15%

Iron 8%

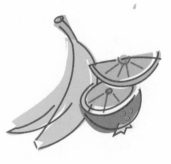

Orange Mango Magnificence™

1 cup oranges

½ cup bananas

1 cup mangos

1 cup orange sherbet

½ cup ice

. . . .

Nutritional Information

Calories 570   Calories from fat 45

Total fat 5 g   7%

Saturated fat 2.5 g   13%

Cholesterol 10 mg   4%

Sodium 100 mg   4%

Total carbohydrates 135 g   45%

Dietary fiber 5 g   19%

Sugars 114 g

Protein 4 g

Vitamin A 130%

Vitamin C 100%

Calcium 15%

Iron 4%

Orange Oomph™

1 cup orange juice

1 cup strawberries

½ cup blueberries

1 cup pineapple sherbet

½ cup ice

. . . .

Nutritional Information

Calories 430   Calories from fat 30

Total fat 3 g   5%

Saturated fat 1 g   6%

Cholesterol 5 mg   2%

Sodium 50 mg   2%

Total carbohydrates 98 g   33%

Dietary fiber 3 g   10%

Sugars 77 g

Protein 5 g

Vitamin A 15%

Vitamin C 360%

Calcium 15%

Iron 6%

Orange Opulence™

1 cup orange juice

1 cup pineapples

½ cup bananas

1 cup lime sherbet

½ cup ice

. . . .

Nutritional Information

Calories 490   Calories from fat 30

Total fat 3.5 g   6%

Saturated fat 1.5 g   8%

Cholesterol 10 mg   3%

Sodium 10 mg   0%

Total carbohydrates 113 g   38%

Dietary fiber 5 g   18%

Sugars 106 g

Protein 5 g

Vitamin A 15%

Vitamin C 260%

Calcium 10%

Iron 8%

Orange Rage™

1 cup orange juice

½ cup bananas

1 cup strawberries

1 cup nonfat vanilla frozen yogurt

½ cup ice

. . . .

Nutritional Information

Calories 410   Calories from fat 15

Total fat 1.5 g   3%

Saturated fat 0 g   0%

Cholesterol 5 mg   1%

Sodium 135 mg   6%

Total carbohydrates 91 g   30%

Dietary fiber 3 g   12%

Sugars 77 g

Protein 13 g

Vitamin A 10%

Vitamin C 360%

Calcium 40%

Iron 8%

Pacific Passion™

1 cup passion fruit/mango juice

1 cup strawberries

½ cup peaches

1 cup pineapple sherbet

½ cup ice

. . . .

Nutritional Information

Calories 460   Calories from fat 25

Total fat 2.5 g   4%

Saturated fat 1 g   6%

Cholesterol 5 mg   2%

Sodium 60 mg   3%

Total carbohydrates 104 g   35%

Dietary fiber 3 g   12%

Sugars 88 g

Protein 4 g

Vitamin A 20%

Vitamin C 170%

Calcium 15%

Iron 6%

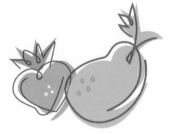

Papa's Pineapple Paradise™

1 cup pineapple juice

1 cup bananas

½ cup peaches

¼ cup coconut

1 cup orange sherbet

½ cup ice

. . . .

Nutritional Information

Calories 580   Calories from fat 100

Total fat 11 g   17%

Saturated fat 9 g   47%

Cholesterol 5 mg   2%

Sodium 125 mg   5%

Total carbohydrates 117 g   39%

Dietary fiber 7 g   29%

Sugars 93 g

Protein 7 g

Vitamin A 25%

Vitamin C 140%

Calcium 6%

Iron 4%

Pineapple Pacify™

1 cup pineapple juice

1 cup pears

½ cup peaches

1 cup orange sherbet

½ cup ice

. . . .

Nutritional Information

Calories 540   Calories from fat 40

Total fat 4.5 g   7%

Saturated fat 2.5 g   12%

Cholesterol 10 mg   4%

Sodium 105 mg   4%

Total carbohydrates 125 g   42%

Dietary fiber 6 g   23%

Sugars 97 g

Protein 3 g

Vitamin A 25%

Vitamin C 130%

Calcium 15%

Iron 4%

Pineapple Pastime™

1 cup pineapple juice

½ cup bananas

1 cup dates

1 cup nonfat vanilla frozen yogurt

½ cup ice

. . . .

Nutritional Information

Calories 880   Calories from fat 15

Total fat 1.5 g   2%

Saturated fat 0.5 g   3%

Cholesterol 5 mg   1%

Sodium 150 mg   6%

Total carbohydrates 216 g   72%

Dietary fiber 15 g   61%

Sugars 190 g

Protein 14 g

Vitamin A 15%

Vitamin C 110%

Calcium 40%

Iron 15%

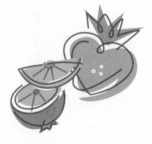

Pineapple Pep™

1 cup pineapple juice

½ cup bananas

1 cup apricots

1 cup orange sherbet

½ cup ice

. . . .

Nutritional Information

Calories 550   Calories from fat 45

Total fat 5 g   8%

Saturated fat 2.5 g   12%

Cholesterol 10 mg   4%

Sodium 105 mg   4%

Total carbohydrates 126 g   42%

Dietary fiber 6 g   23%

Sugars 100 g

Protein 5 g

Vitamin A 100%

Vitamin C 150%

Calcium 15%

Iron 8%

Pineapple Pick-Me-Up™

1 cup pineapple juice

½ cup bananas

1 cup papayas

1 cup pineapple sherbet

½ cup ice

. . . .

Nutritional Information

Calories 490   Calories from fat 20

Total fat 2.5 g   4%

Saturated fat 1.5 g   7%

Cholesterol 5 mg   2%

Sodium 55 mg   2%

Total carbohydrates 113 g   38%

Dietary fiber 5 g   19%

Sugars 98 g

Protein 4 g

Vitamin A 20%

Vitamin C 260%

Calcium 10%

Iron 2%

Pineapple Plantation™

1 cup pineapple juice

1½ cups bananas

2 tablespoons coconut

1 cup pineapple sherbet

½ cup ice

. . . .

Nutritional Information

Calories 630   Calories from fat 60

Total fat 7 g   11%

Saturated fat 6 g   28%

Cholesterol 5 mg   2%

Sodium 90 mg   4%

Total carbohydrates 141 g   47%

Dietary fiber 7 g   27%

Sugars 122 g

Protein 4 g

Vitamin A 15%

Vitamin C 140%

Calcium 8%

Iron 4%

Pomegranate Persuasion™

1 cup pomegranate juice

½ cup pears

1 cup cherries

1 cup nonfat vanilla frozen yogurt

½ cup ice

. . . .

Nutritional Information

Calories 550   Calories from fat 10

Total fat 1.5 g   2%

Saturated fat 0 g   0%

Cholesterol 5 mg   1%

Sodium 140 mg   6%

Total carbohydrates 129 g   43%

Dietary fiber 3 g   12%

Sugars 103 g

Protein 15 g

Vitamin A 8%

Vitamin C 35%

Calcium 40%

Iron 8%

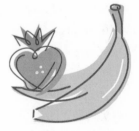

Pomegranate Pom-Poms™

1 cup pomegranate juice

1 cup strawberries

½ cup plums

1 cup raspberry sherbet

½ cup ice

. . . .

Nutritional Information

Calories 490   Calories from fat 40

Total fat 4.5 g   7%

Saturated fat 1 g   6%

Cholesterol 10 mg   3%

Sodium 60 mg   3%

Total carbohydrates 119 g   40%

Dietary fiber 3 g   12%

Sugars 86 g

Protein 6 g

Vitamin A 6%

Vitamin C 90%

Calcium 10%

Iron 6%

Rambunctious Raspberry™

1 cup raspberry juice

1 cup boysenberries

½ cup blueberries

1 cup raspberry sherbet

½ cup ice

. . . .

Nutritional Information

Calories 420   Calories from fat 10

Total fat 1 g   1%

Saturated fat 0 g   0%

Cholesterol 0 mg   0%

Sodium 55 mg   2%

Total carbohydrates 96 g   32%

Dietary fiber 9 g   36%

Sugars 77 g

Protein 4 g

Vitamin A 10%

Vitamin C 170%

Calcium 15%

Iron 40%

Raspberry Royale™

1 cup raspberry juice

1 cup blackberries

½ cup plums

1 cup orange sherbet

½ cup ice

. . . .

Nutritional Information

Calories 470   Calories from fat 45

Total fat 5 g   8%

Saturated fat 2.5 g   12%

Cholesterol 10 mg   4%

Sodium 100 mg   4%

Total carbohydrates 106 g   35%

Dietary fiber 9 g   35%

Sugars 84 g

Protein 5 g

Vitamin A 15%

Vitamin C 170%

Calcium 20%

Iron 40%

Raspberry Rush™

1 cup raspberry juice

1 cup raspberries

½ cup bananas

1 cup nonfat vanilla frozen yogurt

½ cup ice

. . . .

Nutritional Information

Calories 390   Calories from fat 10

Total fat 1.5 g   2%

Saturated fat 0 g   0%

Cholesterol 5 mg   1%

Sodium 140 mg   6%

Total carbohydrates 87 g   29%

Dietary fiber 10 g   41%

Sugars 75 g

Protein 12 g

Vitamin A 8%

Vitamin C 170%

Calcium 40%

Iron 40%

Really . . . Raspberry™

1 cup raspberry juice

1 cup strawberries

½ cup pears

1 cup nonfat vanilla frozen yogurt

½ cup ice

. . . .

Nutritional Information

Calories 350   Calories from fat 10

Total fat 1 g   2%

Saturated fat 0 g   0%

Cholesterol 5 mg   1%

Sodium 140 mg   6%

Total carbohydrates 78g   26%

Dietary fiber 3 g   11%

Sugars 64 g

Protein 12 g

Vitamin A 4%

Vitamin C 240%

Calcium 40%

Iron 40%

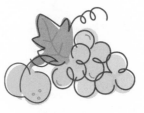

Soy Milk Splash™

1 cup soy milk

1 cup strawberries

½ cup bananas

1 cup vanilla soy-cream

½ cup ice

. . . .

Nutritional Information

Calories 350   Calories from fat 110

Total fat 12 g   19%

Saturated fat 1.5 g   8%

Cholesterol 0 mg   0%

Sodium 210 mg   9%

Total carbohydrates 46 g   15%

Dietary fiber 4 g   15%

Sugars 14 g

Protein 17 g

Vitamin A 4%

Vitamin C 150%

Calcium 10%

Iron 15%

Tangerine Teaser™

1 cup tangerine juice

1 cup apricots

½ cup bananas

1 cup nonfat vanilla frozen yogurt

½ cup ice

. . . .

Nutritional Information

Calories 450   Calories from fat 15

Total fat 2 g   3%

Saturated fat 0 g   0%

Cholesterol 5 mg   1%

Sodium 135 mg   6%

Total carbohydrates 99 g   33%

Dietary fiber 6 g   25%

Sugars 91 g

Protein 14 g

Vitamin A 110%

Vitamin C 170%

Calcium 40%

Iron 10%

Tangerine Trippin'™

1 cup tangerine juice

1 cup bananas

½ cup peaches

1 cup pineapple sherbet

½ cup ice

. . . .

Nutritional Information

Calories 520   Calories from fat 30

Total fat 3 g   5%

Saturated fat 1.5 g   7%

Cholesterol 5 mg   2%

Sodium 45 mg   2%

Total carbohydrates 122 g   41%

Dietary fiber 6 g   25%

Sugars 111 g

Protein 5g

Vitamin A 35%

Vitamin C 160%

Calcium 15%

Iron 6%

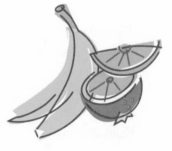

Teeter-Tottering Tangerine™

1 cup tangerine juice

1 cup pineapples

½ cup mangos

1 cup orange sherbet

½ cup ice

. . . .

Nutritional Information

Calories 510   Calories from fat 50

Total fat 5 g   8%

Saturated fat 2.5 g   12%

Cholesterol 10 mg   4%

Sodium 100 mg   4%

Total carbohydrates 118 g   39%

Dietary fiber 4 g   15%

Sugars 102 g

Protein 4 g

Vitamin A 90%

Vitamin C 220%

Calcium 15%

Iron 8%

Temple of Tangerine™

1 cup tangerine juice

1 cup bananas

½ cup papayas

1 cup pineapple sherbet

½ ice

. . . .

Nutritional Information

Calories 510   Calories from fat 30

Total fat 3 g   5%

Saturated fat 1.5 g   7%

Cholesterol 5 mg   2%

Sodium 50 mg   2%

Total carbohydrates 119 g   40%

Dietary fiber 6 g   23%

Sugars 108 g

Protein 5 g

Vitamin A 30%

Vitamin C 220%

Calcium 15%

Iron 6%

Tropical Tease™

1 cup pineapple juice

½ cup bananas

1 cup mangos

1 cup nonfat vanilla frozen yogurt

½ cup ice

. . . .

Nutritional Information

Calories 500   Calories from fat 10

Total fat 1 g   2%

Saturated fat 0 g   0%

Cholesterol 5 mg   1%

Sodium 150 mg   6%

Total carbohydrates 114 g   38%

Dietary fiber 5 g   19%

Sugars 100 g

Protein 11 g

Vitamin A 140%

Vitamin C 190%

Calcium 35%

Iron 4%

Wow! Watermelons™

1 cup watermelon juice

1 cup watermelon

½ cup strawberries

1 cup raspberry sherbet

½ cup ice

. . . .

Nutritional Information

Calories 410   Calories from fat 40

Total fat 4.5 g   7%

Saturated fat 1.5 g   6%

Cholesterol 10 mg   3%

Sodium 60 mg   3%

Total carbohydrates 93 g   31%

Dietary fiber 4 g   15%

Sugars 94 g

Protein 6 g

Vitamin A 40%

Vitamin C 110%

Calcium 15%

Iron 8%

Chapter 6

Fresh-Squeezed Juice Recipes

1. Wash all fruits and veggies first.
2. Cut out bruised areas.
3. Before juicing, remove bitter skins of certain fruits, such as oranges and bananas. Remove stems, leaves, and seeds.
4. After juicing, mix as much pulp back into your drink as you like. Remember, the pulp contains the bulk of the fiber!
5. Drink up right away, as juices spoil rapidly. In a pinch, you can store freshly juiced beverages in an airtight container for twenty-four hours.
6. If using a juicer, be sure to wash it right away, as the pulp will be very difficult to remove later. An old toothbrush and a little elbow grease will work wonders!

Carrot Apple Squeeze™

1 cup carrot juice

1 cup apple juice

. . . .

Nutritional Information

Calories 160   Calories from fat 0

Total fat 0 g   0%

Saturated fat 0 g   0%

Cholesterol 0 mg   0%

Sodium 135 mg   6%

Total carbohydrates 40 g   13%

Dietary fiber 0 g   0%

Sugars 29 g

Protein 1 g

Vitamin A 100%

Vitamin C 15%

Calcium 6%

Iron 0%

Carrot Creation™

1 cup carrot juice

1 cup apple juice

1 ounce ginger juice

. . . .

Nutritional Information

Calories 170   Calories from fat 5

Total fat 0.5 g   1%

Saturated fat 0 g   0%

Cholesterol 0 mg   0%

Sodium 135 mg   6%

Total carbohydrates 44 g   15%

Dietary fiber 0 g   0%

Sugars 29 g

Protein 2 g

Vitamin A 100%

Vitamin C 15%

Calcium 6%

Iron 0%

Carrot Pineapple Poetry™

1 cup carrot juice

1 cup pineapple juice

. . . .

Nutritional Information

Calories 180   Calories from fat 0

Total fat 0 g   0%

Saturated fat 0 g   0%

Cholesterol 0 mg   0%

Sodium 135 mg   6%

Total carbohydrates 41 g   14%

Dietary fiber 0 g   0%

Sugars 24 g

Protein 1 g

Vitamin A 110%

Vitamin C 110%

Calcium 6%

Iron 0%

Carrot Tangerine Machine™

1 cup carrot juice

1 cup tangerine juice

. . . .

Nutritional Information

Calories 160   Calories from fat 10

Total fat 1 g   1%

Saturated fat 0 g   0%

Cholesterol 0 mg   0%

Sodium 125 mg   5%

Total carbohydrates 36 g   12%

Dietary fiber 0 g   0%

Sugars 24 g

Protein 3 g

Vitamin A 120%

Vitamin C 140%

Calcium 10%

Iron 2%

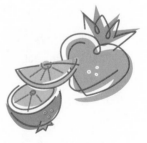

Perfect Carrot Juice™

1 cup carrot juice

1 cup orange juice

. . . .

Nutritional Information

Calories 160   Calories from fat 10

Total fat 1 g   1%

Saturated fat 0 g   0%

Cholesterol 0 mg   0%

Sodium 125 mg   5%

Total carbohydrates 37 g   12%

Dietary fiber 0 g   0%

Sugars 25 g

Protein 3 g

Vitamin A 110%

Vitamin C 220%

Calcium 10%

Iron 2%

Vegetable Vision™

1 cup carrot juice

2 ounces celery juice

1 ounce bell pepper juice

3 ounces tomato juice

2 ounces beet juice

Red onion juice (to taste)

Garlic juice (to taste)

1 chili pepper (your choice)

. . . .

Nutritional Information

Calories 100   Calories from fat 5

Total fat 0.5 g   1%

Saturated fat 0 g   0%

Cholesterol 0 mg   0%

Sodium 560 mg   23%

Total carbohydrates 24 g   8%

Dietary fiber <1 g   3%

Sugars 3 g

Protein 4 g

Vitamin A 120%

Vitamin C 60%

Calcium 10%

Iron 8%

Zestful Carrot Juice™

1 cup carrot juice

½ cup apple juice

½ cup celery juice

. . . .

Nutritional Information

Calories 130   Calories from fat 5

Total fat 0.5 g   1%

Saturated fat 0 g   0%

Cholesterol 0 mg   0%

Sodium 260 mg   11%

Total carbohydrates 32 g   11%

Dietary fiber 0 g   0%

Sugars 15 g

Protein 3 g

Vitamin A 110%

Vitamin C 35%

Calcium 10%

Iron 4%

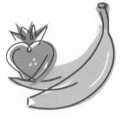

Glossary

Aerobic exercise: An exercise that helps condition your heart and lungs to work harder than normal to supply efficient intakes of oxygen to your muscles.

Anaerobic exercise: An exercise that causes you to use oxygen more rapidly than your body can supply it. "Anaerobic" translates to "without oxygen." Weight training is the best example of anaerobic exercise.

Antioxidant: A chemical compound that slows the process of oxidation. In your body, a vitamin such as beta-carotene, found in many fruits and vegetables, acts as an antioxidant by helping protect your cells from the effects of oxidation (the damage caused by aging, toxins, and pollution).

Beta-carotene: Beta-carotene belongs to the powerful class of phytonutrients known as carotenoids. Carotenoids are proven antioxidants. Beta-carotene, also known as pro–vitamin A, is converted to vitamin A as needed by the body. Vitamin A strengthens the immune system, keeps skin moist and toned, as well as maintains the health of the inner linings of the nose, throat, lungs, intestines, and urinary tract. Vitamin A is absorbed into the bloodstream through dietary fat and is stored in the liver.

Bioflavonoids: Bioflavonoids belong to the class of phytonutrients known as flavones. They help protect the liver from damage from industrial chemicals and viral hepatitis. Bioflavonoids are found in the white rinds of citrus fruits, grapes, plums, black currants, apricots, buckwheat, cherries, blackberries, apples, tea, and onions.

Biotin: A vitamin of the B complex that helps maintain healthy hair, skin, bone marrow, and glands. It also helps produce and transform fatty acids, carbohydrates, and amino acids into energy and is vital to the production of glycogen, an energy source stored in the liver and muscles. Biotin is abundant in eggs, milk products, whole grains, legumes, nuts, yeast, and vegetables in the cabbage family.

Body mass index (BMI): A measurement that helps determine a safe weight for people. Technically, it is your weight (in kilograms), divided by your height (in meters), squared. Generally, a healthy BMI is between 19 and 24. Overweight is a BMI of 25 or more. If your BMI is 30 or more, you would be considered morbidly obese.

Bone density: The basic density, or strength, of your bones.

Cholesterol: A natural chemical compound that is manufactured in the body. Cholesterol is used to build cell membranes as well as brain and nerve tissues. You don't need any extra cholesterol in your diet. Foods from animal products that may contain high amounts of cholesterol include whole-milk dairy products, egg yolks, liver, meat, and some shellfish.

Chromium: A mineral that is instrumental in the release of the hormone insulin that facilitates glucose uptake into cells and energy release.

Chromium picolinate: The essential mineral chromium that has been "chelated," or bonded. This makes it extremely bioavailable, ensuring that it can enter the walls of the body's cells.

Echinacea: A versatile herb used to treat a variety of injuries and illnesses. Internally, it helps to fight bacterial and viral infections, boost the immune system, lower fever, and calm allergic reactions.

Electrolytes: A microscopic ion that cells need to regulate electric charges and flow of water molecules across membranes.

Endorphin: A naturally occurring chemical, or morphine, in your brain that produces relaxing effects.

Essential fatty acids: Lipids, or fats—such as omega-3, omega-6, and omega-9—that are an essential requirement for your body to function properly. We cannot create them on our own, so they are considered "essential" and we get them from our diets.

Fat: A chemical compound consisting of one or more fatty acids. Fat is one of the three most important components of food along with proteins and carbohydrates. Fat is also the primary form in which energy is stored in the body.

Fatty acid: A molecule made mostly of carbon and hydrogen atoms. Fatty acids are the basic foundation of all fats.

Fiber: The part of the food we eat that is actually indigestible. Fiber is important because it stimulates our intestines to move food through our systems and out the back door!

Folic acid: Also known as folate, folic acid is important in the synthesis of DNA, which controls cell functions and heredity as well as tissue growth. Folic acid acts together with vitamin B_{12} in the formation of hemoglobin and red blood cells. Found mostly in the brain and nervous system, folic acid is a vital component of spinal fluid and extracellular fluids, and is an important factor in normalizing functions of the brain.

Free radicals: Free radicals are unstable compounds in your body that are produced when your body burns food into energy. Free radicals can cause serious cell damage linked to diseases such as arthritis and osteoporosis (bone weakening). Free radicals come from all sorts of naturally damaging elements like pesticides, cigarette smoke, drugs, alcohol, sunlight, and pollution.

Fructooligosaccharides (FOS): Fructooligosaccharides are complex carbohydrates that selectively feed friendly intestinal bacteria and impede the growth of harmful bacteria. FOS is a new weapon in the fight against digestive disorders because only recently has technology been able to process and concentrate it from whole foods. Jerusalem artichokes, chicory root, and soybeans are among the most common sources of fructooligosaccharides.

Ginkgo biloba: Ginkgo is a powerful antioxidant, neutralizing harmful free radicals, which can cause many disorders, including premature aging. A member of the Gingkoales family of trees native to southeastern China, it dates back over two hundred million years. The leaves are rich in flavonoids in the fall when they turn from green to yellow, and they hold the healing power of the plant.

Hydrogenated fat: A fat altered by adding hydrogen atoms (see transfatty acid) to increase the shelf life of a product or make it crunchier. Hydrogenated oils, partially hydrogenated oils, vegetable shortenings, and margarines are all hydrogenated fats.

Iodine: A trace mineral primarily received from iodized salt, but also from seafood, seaweed, and vegetables grown in iodine-rich soils. Iodine is necessary for proper function of the thyroid gland and for normal cell function. It keeps skin, hair, and nails healthy and prevents goiter.

Iron: A major mineral found in red meats, liver, egg yolks, peas, beans, nuts, dried fruits, green leafy vegetables, enriched grain products, and liver. Iron is essential to the formation of hemoglobin, the oxygen-carrying factor of the blood that also removes carbon dioxide, and is part of several enzymes and proteins in the body.

Isoflavones, Soy: Part of the class of phytonutrients known as isoflavones, which are derived from soybeans, genistein is regarded as a phytoestrogen. Phytoestrogens are plant-derived hormones similar to the human hormone estrogen that help moderate normal symptoms associated with menopause and promote bone and heart health. Derived from soybeans, soy isoflavones are also considered potent antioxidants capable of reducing LDL cholesterol.

Isometric exercise: A form of exercise that uses your own body for resistance through a series of muscle contractions to build strength.

Lipid: A chemical compound distinguished because it is insoluble in water. Fat and cholesterol are both key members of the larger lipid family.

Lipoprotein: Part of a blood-transporting system made up of chemicals consisting of fat and protein. Lipoproteins with more fat than protein are called low-density lipoproteins (LDLs), or "bad." Lipoproteins with more protein than fat are called high-density lipoproteins (HDLs), or "good." Specifically, lipoproteins are in the blood, functioning mostly to carry cholesterol.

Magnesium: A major mineral or coenzyme vital to metabolism and the entire digestive system. Magnesium also allows the synthesis of sex hormones and the breakdown and resynthesis of proteins; it also strengthens the immune system. In the bloodstream, magnesium helps regulate pH and helps control clotting. Magnesium can be found in many foods, especially green leafy vegetables, beans, nuts, seeds, and grains.

Manganese: Assists, along with enzymes, in the transmission of impulses among the brain, nerves, and muscles and many cell processes. Manganese has also been identified as an antioxidant cofactor, playing a supporting role in the battle against free radicals.

Monounsaturated fatty acid: A fatty acid with one pair of hydrogen atoms missing in the middle of the molecule. Scientifically, the empty space is called an "unsaturation." Monounsaturated fatty acids are good fats, found in edible plants and seafoods. Canola and olive oils are both rich sources of monounsaturated fats. Monounsaturated fatty acids have also been shown to help lower levels of "bad" cholesterol (LDL) in the blood.

Neurotransmitter: A chemical substance such as serotonin that helps transport nerve impulses across a synapse. The boosting of neurotransmitters in your brain can help you feel happier, more relaxed, and even sexier.

Oxidation: Oxidation is simply the process that turns an apple brown soon after you slice into it. In your body oxidation can lead to more rapid aging and cell damage. Scientifically, it is the result of oxygen combining with a chemical substance in which the atoms lose electrons.

Percent Daily Value (%DV): The percentage of daily nutrients recommended by government experts, which has been designed to help us determine the proper amounts of nutrients we should be getting from the foods we eat. Generally, it appears on food labels listed as "Nutritional Facts."

Phytonutrients: Compounds derived from plant, or "phyto," origins that are nutritious or show metabolic biological activity.

Polyunsaturated fatty acid: A fatty acid missing more than one pair of hydrogen atoms. Polyunsaturated fats are found in plant and seafoods. Corn and safflower oils are good sources of polyunsaturated fatty acids. Polyunsaturated fats are somewhat of a mixed blessing as they can help lower levels of both "good" (HDL) cholesterol and "bad" (LDL) cholesterol in the blood.

Psyllium: A gentle fiber that is easily tolerated by children and adults and, being a soluble fiber, is effective in reducing blood cholesterol levels. Psyllium has the greatest bulking activity of any dietary fiber to date, making elimination smoother and more regular, and absorbing toxins on its journey through your system.

RDA and RDI: Recommended Dietary Allowance and Reference Daily Intake are terms to describe the U.S. Department of Agriculture's minimum standards of vitamins and minerals for basic health. The RDAs were established in 1968. The RDIs are more recent.

Resistance training: A means of increasing your muscle strength, power, and endurance using resistance as the method of conditioning: for example, isometric exercises using your own body for resistance and aquatic workouts using the resistance of water to build strength.

Rice protein isolate: Rice may be somewhat low in protein; however, its exceptional balance of amino acids makes the protein of very high quality, so it is more easily absorbed by the body than most grains and cereals, including whole wheat.

Saturated fatty acid: A fatty acid with the very highest number of hydrogen atoms attached to every single carbon atom. In other words, it is *saturated* with hydrogen atoms. Most often, saturated fatty acids are found in animal and dairy products such as whole milk, butter, cheeses, and meats. Saturated fatty acids are considered bad because they can raise levels of "bad" cholesterol (LDL) in the blood. In fact, high levels of LDL cholesterol are a major factor toward the risk of heart disease.

Selenium: A mineral known as a powerful antioxidant, working effectively by itself as well as in conjunction with other antioxidants. Selenium protects the liver from damage; inhibits oxidation of fats; helps maintain a strong immune system; improves assimilation of vitamin E; helps protect the body from damage due to environmental pollution, including blocking the toxic effects of heavy metals such as cadmium and mercury; and helps prevent cancer, heart disease, arthritis, and degenerative changes in the kidneys, liver, and pancreas.

Soy protein isolate: The soybean is the champion protein producer of the legume family. One cup of cooked soybeans delivers 20 grams of protein, plus a good helping of iron. In addition, a growing body of evidence shows that soy protein, because of its high phytonutrient content such as isoflavones, phytosterols, and saponins, lowers the level of "bad" (LDL) cholesterol in the body and thus reduces the risk of heart disease. Soy protein is equivalent to animal proteins in its "rated quality," or its balance of essential amino acids.

Trans-fatty acid: A polyunsaturated fatty acid created during the process of hydrogenation, where some of the missing hydrogen atoms have been put back chemically resulting in "straighter" fatty acids, which then turn back into solids at higher temperatures. Trans-fatty acids are currently being carefully studied to see how they affect levels of "bad" cholesterol (LDL).

Zinc: An essential mineral considered an "enabler" because it helps the body reap maximum benefits from antioxidants. Zinc is necessary for vitamin A to reach full effectiveness and for proper function of the eyes and the neuromuscular system. Zinc maintains taste and smell acuity, normal growth, and sexual development and is important for fetal growth and wound healing.

On-line Resources

The Internet is an extremely valuable tool that can be used as a source of information on a wide range of topics at the touch of your fingertips and the speed of light. The following websites were used as research for this book:

American Academy of Family Physicians

www.aafp.org

The American Academy of Family Physicians represents a group of more than ninety thousand family physicians, family practice residents, and medical students across the country. Since 1947, their mission has been to provide information about the science of family medicine and to ensure high-quality care for all patients.

American Cancer Society

www.cancer.org

The American Cancer Society (ACS) is a community-based voluntary health organization that can be found in cities across America. Headquartered in Atlanta, Georgia, the ACS is dedicated to eliminating cancer as a major health threat by helping to prevent cancer, save more lives, and lessen the suffering from cancer, using research, education, advocacy tools, and service. On their website you can find out all sorts of things such as how you can connect with other survivors and how to cope with a cancer diagnosis.

American Diabetes Association

www.diabetes.org

The American Diabetes Association was founded in 1940 and today it is seen as the nation's leading nonprofit health group that provides diabetes research and information. Their mission is to "prevent and cure diabetes and to improve the lives of all people affected by diabetes." You can find many answers on how to prevent diabetes, as well as helpful hints about nutrition and exercise on their website.

American Dietetic Association
www.eatright.org
The American Dietetic Association (ADA) is America's largest organization of food and nutrition professionals. ADA members, 75 percent of whom are registered dietitians (R.D.s) and 4 percent dietetic technicians, registered (D.T.R.s), represent a wide range of interests, including public health concerns; sports nutrition; diet counseling; cholesterol reduction; diabetes, heart, and kidney disease; vegetarianism; scientific research; and many types of education programs.

American Heart Association
www.americanheart.org
The mission of the American Heart Association (AHA) is to reduce disability and death from cardiovascular diseases and stroke. You can find all sorts of helpful information on their website including the warning signs of strokes, understanding high blood pressure, and the keys to living a healthier lifestyle, to name just a few.

American Obesity Association
www.obesity.org
The American Obesity Association (AOA) was founded to help fight the condition known as obesity that affects more than one-quarter of all adults and one in five children. The effects of obesity are devastating. So the AOA, along with the AOA Research Foundation, were founded to be a catalyst of positive change. To help you better understand obesity and what can be done to change the picture from neglect to action, log on to their website.

Center for Food Safety and Applied Nutrition— Reading Food Labels
vm.cfsan.fda.gov/~lrd/advice.html
An offshoot of the FDA website, here the Center for Food Safety and Applied Nutrition offers great advice for consumers on a wide variety of important topics such as nutrition and weight loss, supplements, food-borne illnesses, food preparation, and much more! In fact, it's a great place to help you read a food label properly.

Center for Science in the Public Interest

www.cspinet.org

The Center for Science in the Public Interest (CSPI) has been help-ing the public better understand the truth about many things that af-fect our lives since 1971. One way they help educate and inform is through their *Nutrition Action Healthletter*. In fact, because of the CSPI's efforts, many important nutritional changes are now in place, for instance, a new federal law is on the books that helps set the standards for health claims on food labels and provides nutritional information on most packaged foods; the CSPI has also encouraged thousands of restaurants to add healthier options to their menus. The CSPI is funded mostly through the eight hundred thousand subscribers to its *National Action Healthletter* and individual donations. The other almost 5 per-cent to 10 percent of the CSPI's annual revenue of $15 million comes from private foundation grants. *Nutrition Action Healthletter* accepts no advertising, and the CSPI accepts no corporate or government grants.

Centers for Disease Control

www.cdc.gov

The Centers for Disease Control and Prevention (CDC) is recognized as the leading federal authority for protecting the health and safety of people here in America as well as overseas. The CDC has been set up to help in the prevention and control of diseases, improve environ-mental health, and promote health through education and activities designed to improve the health of the people of the United States. The main unit of the CDC is located in Atlanta, Georgia, and is an agency of the Department of Health and Human Services.

Food and Drug Administration

www.fda.gov

The Food and Drug Administration (FDA) is one of the nation's oldest and most respected consumer protection agencies. The FDA's mission is to promote and protect the public health by helping safe and effec-tive products reach the market in a timely way, and monitoring prod-ucts for continued safety after they are in use.

Food and Nutrition Information Center

www.nal.usda.gov/fnic/Fpyr/pyramid.html

The Food and Nutrition Information Center (FNIC) is provided as a public service by the National Agricultural Library (NAL), Agricultural Research Service (ARS), and the United States Department of Agriculture (USDA). The above address will take you directly to the Food Guide Pyramid to learn more about it. If you navigate around a bit you will also be able to access information on important topics from A to Z, including aging, AIDS/HIV, emergency preparedness, nutrition assistance programs, supplements, and dozens more.

The National Academies
www.nationalacademies.org
The National Academies are composed of four organizations: the Institute of Medicine, the National Academy of Sciences, the National Academy of Engineering, and the National Research Council. Originally, a congressional charter approved by President Abraham Lincoln in 1863 created the National Academy of Sciences. Under this scientific charter, the National Research Council was founded in 1916, the National Academy of Engineering in 1964, and the Institute of Medicine in 1970.

The National Academy of Sciences was designed by our government to act as a federal adviser on scientific and technological matters. However, the academy and its associated branches are not governmental; the organizations are actually private, so they do not receive direct federal monies for their work.

National Cancer Institute: Eat 5 to 9 a Day for Better Health
5aday.nci.nih.gov
The National Cancer Institute (NCI), a world leader in biomedical cancer research, is the national health authority for the 5 a Day for Better Health Program, dedicated to helping change our behavior and create more effective strategies to increase our fruit and vegetable consumption. This website is super fun, with lots of info and terrific, totally free recipes. The national 5 a Day for Better Health Program gives Americans a simple, positive message—eat five or more servings of fruits and vegetables every day for better health. The program is sponsored jointly by the National Cancer Institute and the Produce for Better Health Foundation (PBH), a nonprofit consumer education foundation that represents the fruit and vegetable industry.

National Institute of Child Health and Human Development

www.nichhd.nih.gov

The National Institute of Child Health and Human Development (NICHHD) is part of the National Institutes of Health, the biomedical research arm of the U.S. Department of Health and Human Services. The mission of the NICHHD is to make sure that every child in America is born healthy and wanted, that women do not suffer any adverse effects from the reproductive process, and that all kids are given the opportunity to fulfill their potential for a healthy and productive life, free of disability or disease.

National Library of Medicine

www.nlm.nih.gov

For more detailed information on various nutritional topics, try the United States National Library of Medicine's website.

Office of the Surgeon General

www.surgeongeneral.gov

The surgeon general of the United States has been the nation's leading spokesperson on matters of public health since 1871. So far, seventeen men and women have served in this key position, including the most recent, Vice Admiral Richard H. Carmona, M.D., M.P.H., F.A.C.S., who was sworn in as surgeon general on August 5, 2002. The surgeon general is the principal adviser on public health and scientific issues.

Supplement Watch

www.supplementwatch.com

Supplement Watch is a privately held corporation that is self-funded. It consists of scientists, nutritionists, physiologists, and other health professionals dedicated to inform and educate on the pros and cons of dietary supplementation. Started in 1999, this group service was formed in response to the growing confusion surrounding the topic of nutrition and dietary supplements.

Tufts Center on Nutrition Communication

navigator.tufts.edu

This is a fun site from the experts at Tufts University, with lots of information and quizzes you can take. It can also be used to help you evaluate other health and nutrition websites with a rating system. In-formation includes topics on everything from men, women, and family concerns to seniors' issues, weight management, and hot topics such as sports nutrition and food safety.

U.S. Department of Agriculture
www.usda.gov
President Abraham Lincoln founded the U.S. Department of Agriculture (USDA) in 1862 to be a resource and guide for all that he called the "people's department." Back then, 48 percent of all Americans were farmers who needed healthy seeds and good information to grow their crops. Today, the USDA continues Lincoln's legacy by serving all Americans.

In fact, the mission of the USDA is to basically enhance the quality of life for the American people by supporting agriculture in many ways that include: ensuring a safe, affordable, and nutritious food supply for all; caring for lands; supporting practical development of rural communities; and working to reduce hunger in America and throughout the world. In other words, the USDA envisions a healthy and productive nation in harmony with the land.

U.S. Department of Health and Human Services
National Institutes of Health
www.nih.gov
Founded in 1887, the National Institutes of Health (NIH) today is one of the world's foremost medical research centers and the federal focal point for medical research in the United States. The goal of NIH research is to acquire new knowledge to help prevent, detect, diagnose, and treat disease and disability. The mission is to uncover new knowledge that will lead to better health for everyone.

WebMD
webmd.com or aolsvc.health.webmd.aol.com
WebMD is a superfriendly source of health-care information on the Web. Their mission is "to be the most objective, credible and trusted source of consumer healthcare information that helps people play an active role in managing their own health." Just log on and within a few seconds you can easily find information on topics concerning your health and wellness.

On-line Blenders and Juicers

Acme® Juicers

www.juicersdirect.com

There are hundreds of websites besides the one above that offer high-quality Acme juicers at affordable prices; this site is one of my favorites.

Blendtec®

www.blendtec.com

Blendtec is the commercial blender division of a company called K-TEC that started making home grain mills over twenty years ago. Success led to a home bread mixer and then a blender, which proved to be a big hit. As smoothies began getting more popular K-TEC designed a blender for commercial use and soon captured the market by storm.

Omega® Juicers

www.omegajuicers.com

Omega juicers are powerful, priced fairly reasonably, and very easy to use. FYI: The Omega Products family has been doing business from the same factory they started in back in 1958. Considered by many as a leader in the juicing field, they recently introduced their Omega Model 4000 Pulp Ejector that ejects the pulp into a separate container. They also make some great wheat-grass juicers.

Vita-Mix®

www.vitamix.com

Vita-Mix Corporation designs and makes high-quality blenders engineered for terrific durability and versatility.

References

American Cancer Society. "Yes You Can!" Eat 5 a Day. www.cancer.org.

American Heart Association. *An Eating Plan for Healthy Americans: Our American Heart Association Diet*. 2002. www.americanheart.org.

Baillie-Hamilton, Paula, M.D. *The Body Restoration Plan*. New York: Avery Books, 2002.

Balch, James F., M.D., and Phyllis A. Balch, C.N.C. *Prescription for Nutritional Healing*. New York: Avery Books, 2000.

———. *Prescription for Nutritional Healing: A-to-Z Guide to Supplements*. New York: Avery Books, 1998.

Bureau of the Census (U.S.). *Statistical Abstract of the United States: The National Data Book: 1997*,117th ed. Washington, D.C.: Government Printing Office, 1997.

Burke, Edmund, Ph.D. *Optimal Muscle Performance and Recovery*. New York: Avery Books, 1999, 2003.

Burnie, David, et al. *Visual Encyclopedia of Science*. New York: Dorling Kindersley, 2000.

Carper, Jean. *FOOD: Your Miracle Medicine*. New York: HarperCollins, 1993, 1998.

Center for Nutrition Policy and Promotion. "The Food Guide Pyramid, USDA: The Food Groups: Breads, Cereals, Rice, and Pasta." *Home and Garden Bulletin* 252 (August 1992; revised October 1996).

Center for Science in the Public Interest, Nutrition Action Health Letter. *Ten Super Foods You Should Eat*. www.cspinet.org/nah/10foods_good.html.

Chopra, Deepak, M.D. *The Seven Spiritual Laws of Success*. San Rafael, Calif., and Novato, Calif.: Amber-Allen Publishing and New World Library, 1994.

Committee on Military Nutrition Research, Institute of Medicine. *The Role of Protein and Amino Acids in Sustaining and Enhancing Performance*. 1999, Committee Overview, 25.

Gerstenzang, James. "Bush Promotes Fitness, Raises Millions in Florida." *Los Angeles Times,* June 22, 2002, The Nation, 12.

Greenwood-Robinson, Maggie, Ph.D. *20/20 Thinking: 1,000 Strategies to Sharpen Your Mind, Brighten Your Mood, and Boost Your Memory.* New York: Avery Books, 2003.

Grimes, MaDonna, with Jim Rosenthal. *Work It Out.* New York: Avery Books, 2003.

Haas, Elson M., M.D. *Staying Healthy with Nutrition.* Berkeley, Calif.: Celestial Arts Publishing, 1992.

———. *The Staying Healthy Shopper's Guide.* Berkeley, Calif.: Celestial Arts Publishing, 1999, 71.

Hoffmann, Bill. "Cancer Threat for Snackers." *New York Post,* April 26, 2002, all editions, 7.

Horowitz, Janice M. "10 Foods That Pack a Wallop: Staying Healthy." *Time,* January 21, 2002, 76–77.

Jacobson, Michael F., Ph.D., Jayne G. Hurley, R.D., and the Center for Science in the Public Interest. *Restaurant Confidential.* New York: Workman, 2002.

Jamba website: www.jambajuice.com.

Joseph, James A., Ph.D., Daniel A. Nadeau, M.D., and Anne Underwood. *The Color Code: A Revolutionary Eating Plan for Optimum Health.* New York: Hyperion, 2002, 197.

Kolata, Gina. "Vitamins: More May Be Too Many." *New York Times,* Science Desk, April 29, 2003. www.nytimes.com.

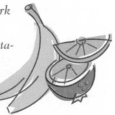

Lieberman, Shari, Ph.D., and Nancy Bruning. *The Real Vitamin & Mineral Book.* New York: Avery Books, 1997.

Mayfield, Eleanor. "A Consumer's Guide to Fats." *FDA Consumer,* May 1994.

Mitchell, Steve. "Trans-Fats Should Be Avoided." *UPI Medical Correspondent, United Press International,* July 11, 2002.

Mokdad, Ali H., et al. "The Continuing Epidemics of Obesity and Diabetes in the United States." *Journal of the American Medical Association,* September 12, 2001, Vol. 286, No. 10, 1195–1200.

National Academy of Sciences, National Center for Chronic Disease Prevention and Health Promotion. *Prescription for Lower Chronic Disease Risk: Less Fat and More Fruits, Vegetables, and Complex Carbohydrates,* March 1, 1989.

National Institutes of Health, Press Release. "Calcium Crisis Affects American Youth." December 10, 2001.

Nelson, Nancy J. "U.S. Department of Health and Human Services, Nurses' Health Study: Nurses Helping Science and Themselves." *Journal of the National Cancer Institute* 92 (April 19, 2000): 597–99.

Nestle, Marion. *Food Politics: How the Food Industry Influences Nutrition and Health.* Berkeley and Los Angeles: University of California Press, 2002, 9.

Nestle, Marion, Ph.D., M.P.H., and Michael F. Jacobson, Ph.D. *U.S. Department of Health and Human Services; Halting the Obesity Epidemic: A Public Health Policy Approach.* Public Health Rep 2000, 115: 12–24, January/February 2000.

Ornish, Dean, M.D. *Dr. Dean Ornish's Program for Reversing Heart Disease.* New York: Ivy Books, 1990, 1996.

———. *Eat More, Weigh Less.* New York: Harpertorch, 1993, 2001.

Physician's Committee for Responsible Medicine, The Cancer Project. *Food as Medicine: The New Four Food Groups.* PCRM is a Washington, D.C.–based nonprofit organization promoting preventative medicine, good nutrition, and higher standards in research. www.cancerproject. org/medicine/nffg.html.

Purba, M., et al. "Skin Wrinkling: Can Food Make a Difference?" *Journal of the American College of Nutrition,* February 2001, 71–80.

Rivas, Paul, M.D. *Turn Off the Hunger Switch Naturally.* New York: Avery Books, 2003.

Rostler, Suzanne. "Whole Grains Can Help Cut Insulin, Cholesterol." *American Journal of Clinical Nutrition* 2002 76 (July 29, 2002): 390–98. www.nlm.nih.gov/medlineplus/news/fullstory_8707.html.

Schlosser, Eric. *Fast Food Nation.* New York: Houghton Mifflin, 2001.

Schorr, Melissa. "Fish Oils Soften Arteries, May Fight Heart Attack," A study partially funded by the drug company F. Hoffmann-La Roche. *American Journal of Clinical Nutrition* 2002 76 (July 31, 2002): 326–30.

Smith, Patricia Burkhart, and Muriel MacFarlane, R.N., M.A., with Eugene Kalnitsky, M.D. *The Complete Idiot's Guide to Wellness.* Indianapolis: Alpha Books, 2002.

Sutherland, Max, and Alice K. Sylvester. *Advertising and the Mind of the Consumer.* Australia: Allen & Unwin, 1993, 2000.

U.S. President's Council on Physical Fitness and Sports. *Physical Activity and Health: A Report of the Surgeon General.* Washington, D.C.: Department of Health and Human Services, 1996.

Warner, Jennifer. "A Drink a Day Keeps Arteries Healthy: Another Heart-Healthy Reason to Drink Alcohol in Moderation." *WebMD Medical News,* May 15, 2003. webcenter.health.webmd.netscape.com/content/article/64/72523.htm.

Weil, Andrew, M.D. *8 Weeks to Optimum Health.* New York: Ballantine, 1997.

Zimlichman, Reuven, M.D. Wolfson Medical Center and Tel Aviv University, Eighteenth Annual Scientific Meeting of the American Society of Hypertension. New York, May 14–16, 2003.

Zwillich, Todd. "U.S. Panel Says No Amount of Trans-Fat Is Safe." Washington, D.C.: Reuters Health, July 11, 2002.

Jamba Juice® Store Locator

For the full Jamba experience, visit your local Jamba Juice store. To find the nearest location, log on to our website at www.jambajuice.com or call 888-JAMBA-12.

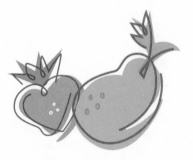

Index

238   Index

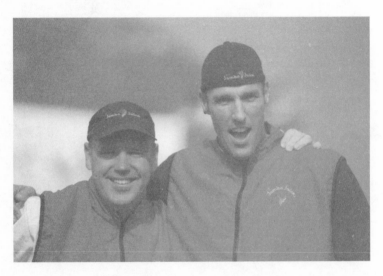

Paul Clayton, CEO, and Kirk Perron, founder of Jamba Juice, after completing the Jamba Juice Wildflower Festival Triathlon at Lake San Antonio, California, in May 2003. Photo courtesy of Mike Larson.